THE CARNIVORE CURE BLUEPRINT:

A Meat -Based Solution to Ultimate Health and Wellness

Ralph S. Phair

Copyright © [2024] [Ralph S. Phair]

All rights reserved.

No part of this book may be reproduced, distributed, or transmitted in any form or by any means, including photocopying, recording, or other electronic or mechanical methods, without the prior written permission of the publisher, except in the case of brief quotations embodied in critical reviews and certain other noncommercial uses permitted by copyright law. For permission requests, write to the publisher at the address below.

Disclaimer:

This book is intended for informational purposes only and does not constitute medical advice. The author is not a licensed medical professional, and readers should consult with a qualified healthcare provider before making any changes to their diet, lifestyle, or health regimen. The author and publisher disclaim any liability for any outcomes resulting from the application of information provided in this book.

Table of Contents

Part 1: Understanding the Carnivore Lifestyle

Introduction: Why Meat?

When I first stumbled upon the idea of a meat-only diet, I laughed. Surely, this was just another extreme trend in a long line of dietary fads, right? I mean, how could eating *only* meat possibly lead to better health? Weren't we supposed to fear red meat, cut back on fat, and pile our plates high with greens? But sometimes, life has a funny way of challenging everything you thought you knew.

This book isn't about following a trend or making headlines. It's about something much deeper: the realization that what we've been told about nutrition might not be the whole truth. It's about rediscovering the power of simplicity, the healing potential of meat, and the joy of eating without fear. Whether you're here out of curiosity, frustration with failed diets, or a deep desire to heal your body, welcome. You're in the right place.

In this introduction, I'll share my personal journey to the carnivore diet, trace the fascinating history of meat in human nutrition, and explain why this book stands apart from the rest. Together, we'll challenge old paradigms, uncover new possibilities, and embark on a journey that could transform your life as it did mine.

My Journey to the Carnivore Diet

I didn't set out to become a champion of the carnivore lifestyle. In fact, my journey started in the same place as many others: confusion, frustration, and a deep desire to feel better.

For years, I followed the conventional advice. I dutifully filled half my plate with vegetables, avoided saturated fats like the plague, and believed that carbs were my body's preferred source of energy. Yet, despite my best efforts, I felt worse with each passing year. My energy levels were non-existent. My weight yo-yoed unpredictably. And worst of all, I battled chronic inflammation that no doctor seemed able to explain.

At some point, I hit rock bottom. I remember sitting in a doctor's office, holding a list of prescriptions that felt more like a prison sentence than a solution. There had to be another way. That's when I started to question everything I thought I knew about health.

My initial foray into alternative diets led me to keto, and while I saw some improvements, something still wasn't quite right. It was during a late-night internet rabbit hole that I first stumbled upon the carnivore diet. The testimonials seemed too good to be true: weight loss, mental clarity, freedom from chronic pain. Could it really be that simple?

Skeptical but desperate, I decided to try it for 30 days. The first week was rough—headaches, fatigue, and an intense longing for anything resembling bread. But then something shifted. My energy came roaring back. My inflammation began to fade. And for the first time in years, I felt truly *alive*.

That 30-day experiment turned into a lifestyle, and the rest is history. The carnivore diet didn't just change my health; it changed my perspective on food, nutrition, and what it means to thrive. Now, I'm here to share what I've learned so you can experience the same transformation.

The Evolution of Meat-Based Nutrition

To understand why the carnivore diet works, we need to go back—way back—to the very beginning of human history.

Our ancestors didn't have the luxury of supermarkets, fad diets, or even the concept of "balanced" meals. Their survival depended on one thing: eating what was available. And for most of human history, that meant meat.

Archaeological evidence shows that early humans were skilled hunters, relying on large animals for sustenance. Meat provided the dense nutrition they needed to fuel their brains, build strong bodies, and endure harsh environments. The advent of tools and fire only amplified this, allowing our ancestors to extract even more nutrients from their prey.

But here's the thing: this wasn't just about survival. Meat wasn't a fallback plan; it was the foundation of human evolution. The high-fat, high-protein diet of our ancestors played a critical role in the development of our large brains and advanced cognitive abilities. Without meat, we wouldn't be the humans we are today.

Fast forward to the modern era, and things have changed dramatically. The agricultural revolution shifted our diets toward grains and plant-based foods. While this allowed civilizations to grow, it also introduced new health challenges, from nutrient deficiencies to chronic diseases.

Today, we live in a world dominated by processed foods, sugar, and dietary misinformation. We've been told to fear meat, avoid fat, and prioritize carbohydrates. But what if the key to reclaiming our health lies in returning to our roots? What if meat—long vilified by modern nutrition—holds the answers we've been searching for?

In this book, we'll explore how embracing a meat-based diet can help us reconnect with our evolutionary heritage, heal our bodies, and thrive in ways we never thought possible.

What Makes This Book Different

By now, you might be wondering: *Why another book on the carnivore diet?* It's a fair question. There are plenty of resources out there, but here's why this one is worth your time.

First, this book isn't just about theory; it's about practicality. While many books focus on the "why," I'm equally committed to the "how." You'll find detailed meal plans, grocery lists, and troubleshooting tips to make your transition to carnivore as seamless as possible.

Second, I've taken the time to address the controversies and criticisms head-on. The carnivore diet isn't without its detractors, and I believe in providing a balanced, evidence-based perspective. Whether it's concerns about sustainability, nutrient deficiencies, or the ethics of meat consumption, we'll tackle it all with honesty and transparency.

Third, this book is deeply personal. I'm not a scientist or a celebrity chef; I'm someone who has lived the journey. I've faced the challenges, reaped the rewards, and learned countless lessons along the way. My goal is to share these insights in a way that's relatable, inspiring, and actionable.

Finally, this book goes beyond food. While nutrition is the cornerstone of the carnivore diet, it's not the whole story. We'll also explore how this lifestyle impacts your mental health, relationships, and overall quality of life. The carnivore cure isn't just about what you eat; it's about how you live.

So, whether you're a seasoned carnivore, a curious skeptic, or someone at their wit's end with traditional diets, this book has something for you. Together, we'll uncover the truth about meat, challenge the status quo, and embark on a journey toward optimal health and vitality.

Welcome to The Carnivore Cure. Let's get started.

The Science Behind Meat-Based Nutrition

The human body is a marvel of biological engineering, and its relationship with food is both complex and fascinating. At the heart of this relationship lies the simple truth: what we eat profoundly impacts how we function, heal, and thrive.

For decades, we've been bombarded with mixed messages about nutrition. Carbs are good; carbs are bad. Fat is the enemy; fat is essential. And meat? Depending on who you ask, it's either the ultimate superfood or a ticking time bomb. But when we strip away the noise and focus on the fundamentals, one thing becomes clear: meat provides the most complete and bioavailable nutrition for the human body.

In this chapter, we'll explore the science behind meat-based nutrition, focusing on the role of macronutrients, how meat fuels our body, and the myths that have unfairly tarnished its reputation.

Understanding Macronutrients: Protein, Fat, and Zero Carbs

Protein: The Building Block of Life

Protein is the cornerstone of every cell, tissue, and organ in your body. It's not just about muscles—although it plays a crucial role there, too. Protein is involved in everything from repairing tissues and producing enzymes to supporting immune function and maintaining healthy skin, hair, and nails.

Meat is an unparalleled source of high-quality protein. Unlike plant-based proteins, which often lack one or more essential amino acids, animal proteins are "complete," meaning they provide all the amino acids your body needs.

Fat: The Body's Preferred Fuel

For years, dietary fat was demonized, blamed for everything from obesity to heart disease. But science has since redeemed fat, showing that it's not only essential but also highly beneficial—especially when it comes from animal sources.

Fat provides more than twice the energy per gram compared to carbohydrates or protein, making it an incredibly efficient fuel source. It's also critical for hormone production, brain health, and the absorption of fat-soluble vitamins like A, D, E, and K.

Animal fats, particularly from grass-fed sources, are rich in beneficial compounds like conjugated linoleic acid (CLA) and omega-3 fatty acids, which have anti-inflammatory and heart-protective properties.

Carbohydrates: Not as Essential as You Think

Here's the kicker: while protein and fat are essential macronutrients (meaning your body can't produce them on its own), carbohydrates are not. The human body can function perfectly well—if not optimally—on a diet devoid of carbs.

When you eliminate carbohydrates, your body shifts into a metabolic state called ketosis, where it burns fat for fuel instead of glucose. This not only supports steady energy levels but also reduces inflammation, stabilizes blood sugar, and promotes fat loss.

How Meat Fuels the Body: Energy, Recovery, and Hormones

Energy: The Fat Advantage

One of the most remarkable aspects of the carnivore diet is its ability to provide consistent, long-lasting energy. Unlike carb-heavy diets, which cause energy spikes and crashes, a meat-based diet stabilizes blood sugar and provides a steady fuel supply.

This is because fat metabolism is more efficient and sustainable than carbohydrate metabolism. When you're running on fat, you avoid the rollercoaster of insulin spikes and enjoy a level of mental clarity and physical endurance that's hard to achieve on a standard diet.

Recovery: Healing from the Inside Out

Meat isn't just fuel; it's medicine. The high-quality protein and fat found in animal products are critical for repairing tissues, reducing inflammation, and supporting overall recovery.

For athletes and active individuals, the benefits are even more pronounced. Protein supports muscle repair and growth, while fat provides the energy needed for sustained performance. And because the carnivore diet eliminates inflammatory foods like sugar and grains, it creates an environment where the body can truly heal.

Hormones: Balancing the Body's Messengers

Hormones control nearly every function in your body, from metabolism and energy levels to mood and reproduction. And guess what? They're made from fat and cholesterol.

A meat-based diet provides the raw materials your body needs to produce and regulate hormones effectively. This can lead to improved mood, better sleep, and enhanced fertility—benefits that are often overlooked in discussions about the carnivore diet.

Debunking Myths: Is Meat Really Bad for You?

The war on meat has been raging for decades, fueled by outdated studies, media sensationalism, and a growing push toward plant-based diets. Let's set the record straight by addressing some of the most common myths about meat.

Myth 1: Meat Causes Heart Disease

The idea that saturated fat and cholesterol cause heart disease is based on flawed science from the mid-20th century. Recent research has debunked this claim, showing no significant link between dietary cholesterol and heart disease.

In fact, the real culprits are often sugar and processed foods, which contribute to inflammation, insulin resistance, and arterial damage. Meat, particularly when sourced responsibly, is not the enemy—it's part of the solution.

Myth 2: Meat is Bad for the Environment

While it's true that industrial farming practices can have negative environmental impacts, the story isn't as black-and-white as it's often portrayed. Regenerative agriculture, which focuses on sustainable grazing practices, can actually improve soil health, sequester carbon, and support biodiversity.

The key is choosing high-quality, responsibly sourced meat and supporting farming practices that prioritize sustainability.

Myth 3: You'll Miss Out on Nutrients Without Plants

One of the biggest misconceptions about the carnivore diet is that it lacks essential nutrients. The truth? Meat is one of the most nutrient-dense foods on the planet.

From iron and zinc to B vitamins and omega-3s, animal products provide a wide array of essential nutrients in forms that are more bioavailable than their plant-based counterparts. For example, the iron in spinach is far less absorbable than the heme iron found in red meat.

Why Other Diets Fail

When it comes to dieting, failure is not the exception—it's the rule. Studies show that most diets have a dismal long-term success rate, with people often regaining the weight they lost and then some. The problem isn't necessarily a lack of willpower or motivation; it's that many diets are fundamentally flawed.

Whether it's the complexity of calorie counting, the unsustainable restrictions, or the outright misinformation, most diets fail because they ignore one critical factor: human biology. Our bodies are designed to thrive on simplicity and efficiency, and when we work against those principles, the results are predictable.

Let's dive into the common reasons other diets fail and explore why a carnivore diet addresses these shortcomings.

The Pitfalls of Plant-Based and Mixed Diets

Plant-based diets, whether vegetarian or vegan, are often marketed as the ultimate path to health and sustainability. But behind the glossy brochures and celebrity endorsements lies a stark reality: these diets are riddled with challenges that make them unsustainable for many people.

Nutrient Deficiencies

Plants simply can't compete with meat when it comes to nutrient density. While they provide fiber and certain vitamins, they lack key nutrients like vitamin B12, heme iron, and essential fatty acids. These are crucial for brain function, energy levels, and overall health, and they're only found in significant quantities in animal products.

For example, vegans often have to rely on supplements to avoid deficiencies. But doesn't that defeat the purpose of eating "natural" foods? A diet that requires lab-made pills to sustain basic health might not be as ideal as it's made out to be.

Anti-Nutrients in Plants

Plants come with their own defense mechanisms, including anti-nutrients like oxalates, lectins, and phytates. These compounds can interfere with the absorption of minerals, irritate the gut lining, and contribute to inflammation.

For instance, spinach is often touted as a great source of calcium and iron, but it's also high in oxalates, which bind to these minerals and make them less available to the body. So while you may think you're getting the nutrients you need, your body might tell a different story.

Satiation and Cravings

Another major issue with plant-based diets is their inability to satisfy hunger in the long term. High-carb, low-fat meals can lead to blood sugar spikes and crashes, leaving you hungry, irritable, and reaching for the nearest snack. This constant cycle of hunger and cravings is exhausting and unsustainable.

Mixed diets, which try to combine plant-based foods with some animal products, fare a little better but often fall into the same trap: too many carbs, too little fat, and a reliance on processed foods to fill the gaps.

The Problem with Processed Foods and Sugar

Processed foods and sugar are the true villains of modern nutrition. They're ubiquitous, addictive, and devastating to our health. And yet, they're a staple in nearly every diet that isn't specifically designed to avoid them.

Why Processed Foods Are So Addictive

The food industry has mastered the art of making products that hijack our brain's reward system. By combining sugar, fat, and salt in precise proportions, they create foods that are nearly impossible to resist. This phenomenon, known as "hyper-palatability," is why you can eat an entire bag of chips without feeling satisfied.

But these foods do more than just make us overeat—they actively harm our bodies. Loaded with artificial ingredients, seed oils, and empty calories, processed foods contribute to inflammation, insulin resistance, and a host of chronic diseases.

The Sugar Epidemic

Sugar deserves its own special mention because it's not just a harmless sweetener—it's a metabolic disaster. Excess sugar consumption has been linked to obesity, type 2 diabetes, heart disease, and even mental health issues like anxiety and depression.

One of the biggest problems with sugar is its sneaky nature. It's hidden in everything from salad dressings to so-called "health bars," making it almost impossible to avoid unless you're actively trying to eliminate it.

And let's not forget its addictive properties. Sugar lights up the same pleasure centers in the brain as drugs like cocaine, creating a cycle of dependence that's hard to break.

The Role of Carbs in Processed Foods

Most processed foods are also loaded with refined carbohydrates, which are quickly broken down into sugar in the body. This leads to rapid blood sugar spikes, followed by crashes that leave you tired, hungry, and craving more carbs.

Over time, this cycle wreaks havoc on your metabolism, contributing to weight gain, insulin resistance, and inflammation. It's no wonder so many diets fail when they rely on these foods as staples.

The Elimination Advantage of Carnivory

So, what makes the carnivore diet different? At its core, it's an elimination diet that strips away all the problematic foods that contribute to poor health, leaving only what your body truly needs: nutrient-dense, bioavailable animal products.

A Simple and Sustainable Approach

One of the biggest advantages of the carnivore diet is its simplicity. There's no need to count calories, track macros, or decipher confusing food labels. You eat meat when you're hungry and stop when you're full.

This simplicity is not just freeing—it's also more in tune with how humans are designed to eat. Our ancestors didn't have spreadsheets or calorie calculators; they ate the foods that were available and thrived.

Nutrient Density at Its Best

Meat is nature's multivitamin. It provides everything your body needs to function optimally, from high-quality protein and healthy fats to essential vitamins and minerals. And because these nutrients are in their most bioavailable forms, your body can absorb and use them far more efficiently than anything you'd get from plants or supplements.

Healing Through Elimination

By eliminating inflammatory foods like sugar, grains, and seed oils, the carnivore diet creates an environment where the body can heal. Many people report dramatic improvements in conditions like autoimmune diseases, digestive issues, and chronic pain after adopting a meat-based diet.

This isn't surprising when you consider the role of inflammation in chronic disease. By removing the foods that contribute to inflammation, you give your body a chance to recover and thrive.

The End of Cravings

Perhaps one of the most surprising benefits of the carnivore diet is the way it eliminates cravings. Without the blood sugar rollercoaster caused by carbs and sugar, you'll find yourself feeling full and satisfied after meals.

This makes it much easier to stick to the diet long-term, as you're not constantly battling hunger or cravings. And because the diet is naturally high in fat, you'll have plenty of energy to fuel your day.

Without the distractions of nutrient-poor foods and the constant battle against cravings, the carnivore diet allows you to focus on what really matters: living your life to the fullest. It's not just about surviving—it's about thriving.

The Meat-Based Diet Spectrum

The carnivore diet, with its emphasis on animal products, has emerged as a popular and powerful approach to health. However, within the broader category of meat-based nutrition, there are different variations and adaptations that people follow. While all of them share the core principle of focusing on animal-derived foods, they differ in their inclusivity of other food groups and their approach to macronutrient balance. In this chapter, we'll explore the meat-based diet spectrum, from the strict carnivore approach to hybrids that incorporate a small amount of plant-based foods. Understanding these variations will help you find the diet that best suits your needs, preferences, and health goals.

Strict Carnivore vs. Keto-Carnivore

Strict Carnivore Diet

The strict carnivore diet is exactly what it sounds like: an all-meat, animal-based approach to nutrition. It's the most restrictive of all the meat-based diets and eliminates all plant foods, including fruits, vegetables, nuts, seeds, and even spices that aren't derived from animals. The idea is to consume only animal products—beef, pork, chicken, fish, and animal fats—on a daily basis.

The strict carnivore diet aims to provide the body with everything it needs through nutrient-dense animal foods. This means high-quality proteins, healthy fats, and essential vitamins and minerals that are found in abundance in meat. Proponents of this approach believe that by eliminating all plant-based foods, you can eliminate the many anti-nutrients and irritants that can interfere with digestion and overall health.

For many, the strict carnivore diet can lead to significant health benefits. People report improvements in autoimmune conditions, digestive issues, mental clarity, and weight loss. The simplicity of the diet is also a major draw for those who struggle with decision fatigue and meal planning. With a strict carnivore diet, there's no need to count calories, track macros, or measure food portions. You eat meat until you're full and stop when you're satisfied.

However, there are some challenges with this approach. It's difficult to sustain for some individuals due to its extreme nature. Social situations, dining out, and family meals can become complicated, and the lack of variety may lead to feelings of monotony. Additionally, the diet can be restrictive for those who enjoy plant-based foods or are concerned about the potential long-term effects of eliminating all plant nutrients.

Keto-Carnivore Diet

The keto-carnivore diet is a hybrid between the carnivore and ketogenic diets. It follows the same principles as the strict carnivore diet but with a few adjustments to incorporate the ketogenic approach to fat intake. The primary difference is that, while the strict carnivore diet is focused on consuming primarily protein and fat, the keto-carnivore diet places more emphasis on the high-fat aspect of the ketogenic diet.

In a keto-carnivore diet, the goal is to maintain a state of ketosis—where the body burns fat for fuel instead of carbohydrates—while still adhering to the carnivore principle of consuming animal products. This means that individuals following the keto-carnivore diet will often prioritize fatty cuts of meat (such as ribeye steak, fatty pork belly, and lamb) and may also include high-fat animal products like butter, ghee, and heavy cream.

The keto-carnivore diet is appealing to those who want to reap the benefits of both ketosis and a meat-based approach to nutrition. Like the strict carnivore diet, the keto-carnivore diet eliminates carbohydrates entirely, which can lead to weight loss, improved energy levels, and enhanced mental clarity. However, the added emphasis on fats makes this approach more sustainable for some individuals. The higher fat content helps to maintain energy levels throughout the day and can keep hunger at bay for longer periods of time.

However, there are challenges with this diet as well. Achieving the proper macronutrient balance can be tricky, especially when trying to ensure that the body stays in ketosis. It's easy to overconsume protein, which can interfere with ketosis, or under consume fat, which can leave you feeling hungry or fatigued. Like the strict carnivore diet, the keto-carnivore approach can be restrictive and may not be sustainable for everyone, especially in social or family settings.

Understanding Omnivore-Carnivore Hybrids

What is an Omnivore-Carnivore Hybrid?

The omnivore-carnivore hybrid diet is a more flexible version of the carnivore diet that allows for a small number of plant-based foods alongside animal products. While the strict carnivore diet excludes all plant foods, the omnivore-carnivore hybrid incorporates some vegetables, fruits, and other plant-based items, often for their nutritional benefits or to make the diet more sustainable and enjoyable.

For example, some individuals on an omnivore-carnivore hybrid diet may include low-carb vegetables such as leafy greens, broccoli, and cauliflower. These vegetables are rich in fiber, vitamins, and minerals that support digestion and overall health. Others may include small amounts of berries, nuts, or seeds, which can provide antioxidants and healthy fats. However, the core of the diet remains animal products, with plant foods playing a supporting role rather than being the main focus.

The omnivore-carnivore hybrid diet offers a compromise for those who want the benefits of a meat-based diet but aren't ready to give up plant foods entirely. It's also a good option for those who are new to the carnivore approach and want to ease into it gradually. The inclusion of some plant foods can make the diet more palatable and easier to sustain in the long term.

The Benefits of Omnivore-Carnivore Hybrids

One of the main advantages of the omnivore-carnivore hybrid diet is its flexibility. By allowing a small amount of plant-based foods, it makes the diet more accessible and adaptable to different lifestyles. For example, someone who follows a strict carnivore diet might find it difficult to eat out at restaurants or attend social gatherings where only plant-based options are available. However, by allowing a small amount of plant foods, the omnivore-carnivore hybrid diet offers more variety and options without sacrificing the core principles of meat-based nutrition.

Additionally, some individuals may find that the inclusion of certain plant foods helps them feel more satisfied or reduces cravings. Vegetables like leafy greens can add bulk to meals, making them feel more filling, while fruits can satisfy a sweet tooth without relying on processed sugars. These additions can make the diet more enjoyable and less monotonous, which can help improve adherence in the long term.

Finding Your Perfect Fit

When it comes to choosing a meat-based diet, there is no one-size-fits-all approach. Each person has unique needs, preferences, and health goals, and the key to success is finding the diet that works best for you. Here are a few steps to help you navigate the meat-based diet spectrum and find your perfect fit.

Step 1: Understand Your Goals

Before deciding on a specific meat-based diet, it's important to clarify your goals. Are you looking to lose weight, improve your mental clarity, manage a health condition, or simply feel better overall? Your goals will guide your decision on whether to follow a strict carnivore diet, a keto-carnivore diet, or an omnivore-carnivore hybrid.

For example, if weight loss is your primary goal, the strict carnivore or keto-carnivore diets may be the most effective options, as they promote fat burning and appetite control. On the other hand, if you're looking to improve overall health and are willing to include a small amount of plant foods, an omnivore-carnivore hybrid might be the right fit for you.

Step 2: Experiment and Listen to Your Body

Once you've identified your goals, it's time to experiment with different variations of the carnivore diet. Start by trying a strict carnivore diet for a few weeks and pay attention to how your body responds. Do you feel more energized, clear-headed, and satisfied? Or do you struggle with hunger, fatigue, or digestive issues? If the strict carnivore approach feels too restrictive or unsustainable, try incorporating a small amount of plant foods to see if that helps you feel better.

Listening to your body is key when it comes to finding the right diet for you. Everyone's body is different, and what works for one person may not work for another. Don't be afraid to make adjustments along the way and find the approach that best supports your health and well-being.

Step 3: Consider Sustainability

Sustainability is a critical factor in choosing a diet that will work for you in the long term. The carnivore diet, whether strict or hybrid, can be highly effective, but it may not be the easiest diet to follow forever. Consider how easy it is to maintain the diet in your everyday life, especially in social situations, at family meals, or when dining out. If you find that the strict carnivore diet is too restrictive for you, a keto-carnivore or omnivore-carnivore hybrid may be a more sustainable option.

Part 2: The Carnivore Cure in Action

How to Get Started

The journey into a meat-based diet is one that's exciting, transformative, and, for many, a little intimidating. Whether you're drawn to the carnivore diet for its health benefits, simplicity, or the promise of better energy and mental clarity, it's important to approach the transition thoughtfully. In this chapter, we'll explore the steps to getting started with the carnivore diet, how to transition from your current eating habits, how to prepare your kitchen for the change, and what you can expect as your body adjusts.

Transitioning from Your Current Diet

1. Understanding Your Current Eating Habits

Before diving headfirst into the carnivore diet, it's essential to take a step back and reflect on your current eating habits. What does a typical day of eating look like for you? Do you eat mostly plant-based foods, or is your diet rich in processed items and carbs? Understanding where you're starting from will give you a clearer picture of what adjustments need to be made and how your body may react to the shift.

For example, if you're coming from a typical Western diet that includes a lot of grains, processed foods, sugars, and starches, the transition to an all-meat approach may be more challenging than if you already consume a high-protein or low-carb diet. By identifying your current eating patterns, you'll be able to tailor your transition to the carnivore diet more effectively.

2. Gradual vs. Immediate Transition

When it comes to transitioning to the carnivore diet, there are two main approaches: the gradual transition and the immediate, "cold turkey" approach. Both have their merits, but which one you choose depends on your preferences, health goals, and how your body typically reacts to dietary changes.

- **Gradual Transition**: For many people, a slow and steady transition works best. This approach allows you to ease into the diet, making small adjustments over time.

Start by eliminating processed foods and refined sugars while increasing your intake of animal-based foods. Slowly reduce carbohydrates, focusing on vegetables and fruits with low glycemic indexes, until you're ready to make the full switch to an all-meat diet.

The gradual approach can help your body adjust to the changes in energy sources. Since your body has likely been running on carbohydrates for years, transitioning slowly can prevent the symptoms of carbohydrate withdrawal, such as fatigue, irritability, and cravings. This method is often recommended for people who have struggled with other diets or who have underlying health conditions like metabolic disorders.

- **Immediate Transition**: On the other hand, some people find that diving straight into the carnivore diet works best for them. They prefer the simplicity and decisiveness of cutting out all plant foods from the get-go. For these individuals, the cold turkey approach can be a powerful way to kickstart their health journey. It's not for everyone, though. Some may experience more intense withdrawal symptoms, including brain fog, fatigue, and cravings in the first few days or weeks.

Ultimately, the best approach is the one that feels right for you. If you're not sure which method to use, you can always start with a gradual transition and switch to a more immediate approach once you feel comfortable.

3. Tracking Your Progress

As you transition into the carnivore diet, it's important to keep track of your progress. This doesn't necessarily mean counting calories or macros (unless that's something you find helpful), but paying attention to how your body feels. Are you experiencing more energy throughout the day? Is your digestion improving? Are you noticing any skin changes, like fewer breakouts or less bloating?

Tracking your progress can help you stay motivated, especially when you experience the inevitable challenges of adapting to a new diet. It also helps you understand how your body responds to the carnivore diet and if any adjustments need to be made along the way.

Pantry Purge: Out with the Old, In with the Meat

One of the most crucial steps in preparing for the carnivore diet is clearing out your pantry. It's time to make space for all the nourishing animal-based foods you'll soon be stocking up on. The process of purging your pantry is not only practical but symbolic—out with the processed foods and sugary snacks that have been a crutch, and in with the nourishing, life-sustaining meat that will fuel your body in a way that aligns with your health goals.

1. Clean Out the Processed Foods

Processed foods are a major culprit in many modern health issues, and when transitioning to a meat-based diet, you'll want to get rid of them completely. Take a good look at your pantry and fridge. Are there chips, crackers, cereal, pasta, canned soups, or anything with a long list of ingredients that you can't pronounce? These foods are typically loaded with sugars, preservatives, and unhealthy fats—none of which have a place in your new way of eating.

This doesn't just mean the obvious junk foods. Even some seemingly "healthy" foods, like low-fat dressings, granola bars, and store-bought bread, often contain added sugars, unhealthy oils, and other non-carnivore-friendly ingredients. The goal is to eliminate anything that could tempt you back into old habits and create space for nutrient-dense, whole animal foods.

2. Stock Up on Quality Animal Products

Once your pantry is cleared out, it's time to fill it back up with high-quality animal products. When starting the carnivore diet, you'll want to make sure you're getting the best sources of protein and fat possible. This means choosing grass-fed beef, wild-caught fish, pasture-raised poultry, and free-range eggs. These options are more nutrient-dense and contain fewer harmful chemicals, pesticides, and hormones than their conventionally farmed counterparts.

Don't forget about animal fats, which are an essential part of the carnivore diet. Stock up on tallow, lard, butter, ghee, and other animal fats to help keep you feeling satisfied and support your energy levels. If you're following a keto-carnivore approach, these fats will be crucial for maintaining ketosis.

You'll also want to have a variety of cuts of meat on hand to keep your meals interesting. Consider getting ground beef, steaks, roasts, organ meats, and bones for bone broth. Organ meats like liver and kidneys are some of the most nutrient-dense foods you can eat, packed with vitamins and minerals that are harder to obtain from muscle meat alone.

3. Create a Carnivore-Friendly Kitchen

Once you've purged your pantry and stocked up on animal products, the next step is to make sure your kitchen is carnivore-friendly. This doesn't just mean filling your fridge with meat—it also means getting the right tools and utensils to make preparing your meals easy and enjoyable.

Invest in high-quality cookware that will allow you to prepare your meats properly. A good set of sharp knives, a cast-iron skillet, a slow cooker, and an air fryer can make meal prep a breeze. If you plan on making bone broth, having a large stockpot or pressure cooker is a must.

What to Expect: Adapting to Carnivore

1. The First Few Days: Carbohydrate Withdrawal

In the first few days of transitioning to the carnivore diet, you'll likely experience some initial discomfort. If you've been consuming a diet high in carbohydrates, your body will go through a process of adjusting to burning fat instead of glucose for energy. This shift is commonly referred to as "carb flu," and it can bring about symptoms like fatigue, headaches, irritability, and cravings for sugary foods.

The good news is that this phase is temporary. Most people start to feel better after a few days or up to a week, as their bodies adapt to ketosis—the state where your body uses fat as its primary fuel source. To ease this transition, make sure you're drinking plenty of water and getting enough electrolytes, such as sodium, potassium, and magnesium. This can help alleviate symptoms like headaches and muscle cramps.

2. Increased Energy and Mental Clarity

After the initial transition period, you'll likely start to notice some significant benefits. Many people report feeling more energized and mentally clear after a few weeks on the carnivore diet. Without the blood sugar crashes that come with carbohydrate consumption, your energy levels become more stable, leading to fewer midday slumps and better focus throughout the day.

Mental clarity is another benefit that many people experience. Without the fogginess caused by excess carbs and sugar, your brain can function at a higher level. Some even describe a feeling of "mental sharpness" or enhanced cognitive function. If you've struggled with brain fog or poor concentration in the past, the carnivore diet can offer a noticeable improvement.

3. Digestive Changes and Skin Improvements

Many people also report improvements in their digestion and skin after adopting the carnivore diet. For those with digestive issues like bloating, gas, or IBS, eliminating plant foods can provide significant relief. The carnivore diet's high protein and fat content supports healthy gut function, while the elimination of fiber and plant-based irritants can reduce inflammation in the gut.

As your digestion improves, you may also notice clearer skin. Acne, eczema, and other skin conditions are often exacerbated by inflammatory foods, and by eliminating these triggers, many people experience smoother, healthier skin. However, it's important to note that some people may experience an initial breakout as their body detoxes, but this is typically temporary.

Choosing Your Cuts: Meat Matters

When embarking on the carnivore diet, one of the most critical aspects to consider is the quality and variety of the meat you consume. While the focus is primarily on animal-based products, not all meats are created equal. The way the animal is raised, the type of meat it produces, and how it is prepared can significantly impact the nutritional value of your meals and your overall health. This chapter will guide you through the process of choosing the right cuts of meat, explain the difference between grass-fed and grain-fed meat, and explore the nutritional benefits of organ meats and bone broth.

Grass-Fed vs. Grain-Fed Meat

The Basics: Grass-Fed and Grain-Fed Differences

The debate between grass-fed and grain-fed meat is one of the most frequently discussed topics when it comes to carnivore nutrition. Understanding the differences between these two types of meat is essential for making the best choices for your health.

- **Grass-Fed Meat**: Grass-fed beef comes from cattle that are raised on pasture and eat a natural diet of grasses and forage. This type of meat tends to be leaner, with a different fatty acid profile compared to grain-fed beef. Grass-fed meat is typically higher in omega-3 fatty acids, conjugated linoleic acid (CLA), and antioxidants like vitamin E. These nutrients are known for their anti-inflammatory properties and potential benefits to heart health. Additionally, grass-fed meat tends to be lower in omega-6 fatty acids, which, when consumed in excess, can contribute to inflammation and other health issues.

- **Grain-Fed Meat**: Grain-fed beef comes from cattle that are typically raised in feedlots and fed a diet of grains, corn, and soy. This type of meat is usually fattier, with a higher content of omega-6 fatty acids. While omega-6s are essential in small amounts, an imbalance of omega-6 to omega-3 can contribute to inflammation and chronic disease. Grain-fed meat is often less nutrient-dense than grass-fed, as the grains used to fatten the cattle can alter the nutritional profile of the meat.

Why Grass-Fed is Better for Carnivores

For those following the carnivore diet, the focus should be on nutrient-dense foods that support optimal health. Grass-fed meat offers a superior nutritional profile due to its higher levels of healthy fats and antioxidants. The omega-3s found in grass-fed beef are especially important, as they support brain function, reduce inflammation, and improve cardiovascular health.

In addition, grass-fed meat often contains fewer harmful compounds like pesticides, hormones, and antibiotics, which are commonly found in conventionally raised grain-fed meat. If you're committed to eating as clean and natural as possible, grass-fed meat is a better choice for your carnivore journey.

The Cost of Grass-Fed Meat

One of the most significant drawbacks of grass-fed meat is its cost. Grass-fed beef and other pasture-raised meats are often more expensive than grain-fed varieties due to the way the animals are raised. Grass-fed cattle require more land, time, and care, which results in higher production costs. However, for those committed to improving their health and getting the most nutritional benefit from their meat, the extra cost is often worth it. You can also offset the cost by purchasing in bulk or finding local farms that offer direct-to-consumer sales, which can be more affordable than store-bought options.

Beef, Lamb, Pork, and Beyond: Which to Prioritize

Beef: The Foundation of Carnivore

Beef is often considered the cornerstone of the carnivore diet, and for good reason. It's a versatile meat that provides high-quality protein, healthy fats, and essential nutrients. When selecting beef, opt for a variety of cuts to ensure you're getting a balance of nutrients. Some of the best cuts for the carnivore diet include:

- **Ribeye**: Known for its marbling, ribeye is a fatty cut that provides plenty of energy and satisfaction. It's one of the most nutrient-dense cuts, offering a good amount of protein, healthy fats, and vitamins.

- **Sirloin**: A leaner cut than ribeye, sirloin is still rich in protein and can be a great option for those looking to balance their fat intake. It's a versatile cut that can be grilled, pan-seared, or roasted.

- **Ground Beef**: Ground beef is an affordable and easy-to-prepare option that can be used in a variety of dishes. Opt for higher-fat ground beef, such as 80/20 or 85/15, to ensure you're getting enough fat in your diet.

- **Brisket**: This cut is perfect for slow cooking or smoking, making it a favorite among carnivores. It's a tougher cut that benefits from long, slow cooking, resulting in tender, flavorful meat.

Beef is an excellent source of essential amino acids, iron, zinc, and B vitamins. It's also rich in creatine, which supports muscle growth and energy production. For those looking to build muscle or improve athletic performance, beef is a top choice.

Lamb: A Nutrient-Packed Alternative

Lamb is another excellent choice for the carnivore diet. While not as commonly consumed as beef, lamb offers a unique flavor and a rich nutritional profile. It's an excellent source of protein, omega-3 fatty acids, and minerals like zinc and selenium.

Lamb tends to be fattier than beef, making it a great option for those on a high-fat carnivore diet. Cuts like lamb chops, shoulder, and leg are all great choices, offering plenty of flavor and healthy fats. If you're looking for variety in your carnivore meals, lamb is an excellent option to include.

Pork: A Versatile and Flavorful Meat

Pork is often underrated on the carnivore diet, but it can be a fantastic addition to your meals. While it's not as nutrient-dense as beef or lamb, pork is still a good source of protein and fat. Cuts like pork belly, pork shoulder, and bacon are all excellent options for carnivores.

Pork is also a great source of thiamine, a B vitamin that plays a crucial role in energy production and nervous system health. When choosing pork, look for cuts that are higher in fat, as these will provide the most satiety and energy.

Other Meats to Consider

While beef, lamb, and pork are the most common meats on the carnivore diet, there are plenty of other animal-based options to explore. These include:

- **Bison**: Leaner than beef but still packed with protein, bison is a great alternative for those looking to vary their meat choices.
- **Venison**: A lean, wild game meat that's high in protein and low in fat. It's a great choice for those who enjoy game meats.
- **Chicken and Turkey**: While these meats are lower in fat than beef or lamb, they can still be included in a carnivore diet, especially if you focus on fattier cuts like chicken thighs or duck.

By incorporating a variety of meats into your diet, you ensure that you're getting a range of nutrients that support overall health. However, beef, lamb, and pork should remain your primary focus due to their superior nutrient density and availability.

Organ Meats and Bone Broth: Nutritional Powerhouses

The Benefits of Organ Meats

Organ meats, such as liver, kidneys, heart, and spleen, are often overlooked in the modern diet but are some of the most nutrient-dense foods you can consume. These meats are rich in vitamins, minerals, and amino acids that are essential for maintaining optimal health.

- **Liver**: Often referred to as the "king of organ meats," liver is an incredibly nutrient-dense food. It's packed with vitamin A, B vitamins (especially B12), iron, copper, and zinc. Liver is an excellent choice for those on the carnivore diet because it supports energy production, immune function, and brain health.

- **Heart**: While less commonly consumed, heart meat is an excellent source of CoQ10, an antioxidant that supports cardiovascular health. It's also rich in protein, iron, and B vitamins. Beef heart, in particular, is a great option for those looking to add variety to their carnivore meals.

- **Kidneys**: Rich in vitamins A and B12, kidneys are another powerful organ meat. They're particularly high in phosphorus, a mineral that's important for bone health and energy production. Kidney meat is often described as having a stronger flavor, but it can be prepared in various ways to make it more palatable.

The Importance of Bone Broth

Bone broth is another carnivore-friendly food that offers numerous health benefits. Made by simmering bones (often from beef, chicken, or lamb) for hours, bone broth is packed with collagen, gelatin, and amino acids that support joint health, gut health, and skin elasticity.

- **Collagen and Gelatin**: These proteins are vital for maintaining the integrity of your connective tissues, including joints, tendons, and ligaments. Drinking bone broth regularly can help reduce joint pain, improve skin elasticity, and support overall mobility.

- **Amino Acids**: Bone broth contains essential amino acids like glycine, proline, and glutamine, which play a crucial role in gut health and immune function. Glycine, in particular, supports detoxification processes in the body and promotes relaxation and better sleep.

Bone broth is also incredibly versatile—it can be used as a base for soups, stews, or sauces, or simply sipped as a warm, comforting drink. It's an excellent way to get extra nutrients on a carnivore diet, especially if you're not consuming organ meats regularly.

Choosing the right cuts of meat is essential for optimizing your carnivore diet. Whether you prioritize grass-fed beef, lamb, pork, or a variety of other meats, it's important to select high-quality, nutrient-dense options that will support your health goals. Additionally, incorporating organ meats and bone broth into your diet will provide you with powerful nutritional benefits that go beyond what muscle meats alone can offer.

By making informed choices about the meats you eat, you can create a carnivore diet that's not only satisfying but also rich in the nutrients your body needs to thrive. Whether you're a seasoned carnivore or just starting, these choices will help you make the most of your meat-based nutrition journey.

The Carnivore Meal Plan

Transitioning to a carnivore diet is about embracing simplicity while also finding variety within the scope of meat-based eating. This chapter provides practical tools, including sample weekly meal plans, quick recipes for busy days, and advanced cooking techniques to elevate your meals. Whether you're new to this lifestyle or a seasoned carnivore, this guide ensures you stay nourished, satisfied, and inspired.

Sample Weekly Meal Plans

A well-structured meal plan simplifies decision-making and ensures you're meeting your nutritional needs. Below are three sample plans tailored to different levels of carnivore adherence:

1. Strict Carnivore Meal Plan

Focused exclusively on animal-based foods, this plan is ideal for those seeking an elimination diet or addressing specific health concerns.

Day 1

- **Breakfast: Ribeye Steak**
  Ingredients:
  - 1 ribeye steak (10-12 oz)
  - 1 tbsp tallow or ghee
  - Salt to taste

  Instructions:

- o Heat a skillet on high heat and add tallow.
- o Season the steak with salt.
- o Sear the steak for 3-4 minutes per side for medium-rare.

- **Lunch: Ground Beef Patties**

Ingredients:

- o 1 lb ground beef (80/20)
- o 1 tbsp butter
- o Salt to taste

  Instructions:

- o Form the ground beef into two patties.
- o Heat a skillet and cook the patties for 4-5 minutes per side.
- o Top with butter before serving.

- **Dinner: Roasted Chicken Thighs**

Ingredients:

- o 4 chicken thighs
- o 1 tbsp duck fat

- Salt to taste

Instructions:

- Preheat oven to 400°F (200°C).
- Rub chicken thighs with duck fat and salt.
- Roast for 35-40 minutes until skin is crispy.

Day 2

- **Breakfast: Beef Liver**

Ingredients:

- 8 oz beef liver
- 2 tbsp ghee
- Salt to taste

Instructions:

- Heat ghee in a skillet over medium heat.

- Sear liver for 2-3 minutes per side until browned.

- **Lunch: Grilled Lamb Chops**

Ingredients:

- 4 lamb chops
- 1 tbsp olive oil
- Salt to taste

Instructions:

- Preheat a grill or grill pan.
- Rub lamb chops with olive oil and salt.
- Grill for 4 minutes per side for medium.

- **Dinner: Baked Salmon with Bone Broth**

Ingredients:

- 6 oz salmon fillet
- 1 cup bone broth
- Salt to taste

Instructions:

- Preheat oven to 375°F (190°C).

- Place salmon in a baking dish, pour bone broth around it, and bake for 15-20 minutes.

Day 3

- **Breakfast: Scrambled Eggs with Duck Fat**
  Ingredients:
  - 3 eggs
  - 1 tbsp duck fat
  - Salt to taste

  Instructions:
  - Melt duck fat in a skillet over medium heat.
  - Beat eggs, pour into the skillet, and scramble until set.
- **Lunch: Smoked Brisket**
  Ingredients:
  - 8 oz smoked brisket

- Salt to taste

Instructions:

- Reheat brisket in a skillet over low heat or in the oven.

- **Dinner: Pan-Seared Pork Chops**

Ingredients:

- 2 pork chops
- 1 tbsp lard
- Salt to taste

Instructions:

- Heat lard in a skillet over medium-high heat.
- Sear pork chops for 4-5 minutes per side.

Day 4

- **Breakfast: Bacon and Eggs**

Ingredients:

- o 4 slices of bacon
- o 2 eggs

Instructions:

- o Cook bacon in a skillet until crispy, then set aside.
- o Use the bacon grease to fry eggs to your liking.

- **Lunch: Ribeye Steak with Butter**

Ingredients:

- o 1 ribeye steak
- o 2 tbsp butter

Instructions:

- o Sear steak in a hot skillet for 4-5 minutes per side.
- o Top with butter before serving.

- **Dinner: Grilled Chicken Wings**

Ingredients:

- o 10 chicken wings
- o 1 tbsp salt

Instructions:

- Preheat a grill to medium-high heat.
- Grill wings for 15-20 minutes, turning frequently.

Day 5

- **Breakfast: Bone Marrow with Salt**

Ingredients:

- 2 beef marrow bones
- Salt to taste

Instructions:

- Preheat oven to 450°F (230°C).
- Roast marrow bones for 15-20 minutes until the center is soft.

- **Lunch: Lamb Liver**

Ingredients:

- 8 oz lamb liver
- 1 tbsp butter

- Salt to taste

Instructions:

- Heat butter in a skillet over medium heat.
- Sear liver for 2-3 minutes per side.

- **Dinner: Grilled Swordfish**

Ingredients:

- 6 oz swordfish steak
- 1 tbsp olive oil
- Salt to taste

Instructions:

- Rub swordfish with olive oil and salt.
- Grill for 4-5 minutes per side.

Day 6

- **Breakfast: Scrambled Eggs with Steak Bites**

Ingredients:

- 3 eggs
- 4 oz steak, diced
- 1 tbsp butter

Instructions:

- Sear steak bites in butter until browned.
- Add eggs and scramble until set.

- **Lunch: Roasted Duck Legs**

Ingredients:

- 2 duck legs
- Salt to taste

Instructions:

- Preheat oven to 375°F (190°C).
- Roast duck legs for 45-50 minutes.

- **Dinner: Pan-Seared Scallops**

Ingredients:

- 6 large scallops
- 1 tbsp butter

Instructions:

- Heat butter in a skillet over medium-high heat.
- Sear scallops for 2 minutes per side.

Day 7

- **Breakfast: Pork Belly Strips**

Ingredients:

- 6 oz pork belly
- Salt to taste

  Instructions:

- Cook pork belly strips in a skillet over medium heat until crispy.

- **Lunch: Smoked Salmon**

Ingredients:

- 6 oz smoked salmon

  Instructions:

- Serve smoked salmon cold or lightly warmed.

- **Dinner: Grilled Ribeye**
  Ingredients:
    - 1 ribeye steak
    - 1 tbsp butter

  Instructions:
    - Grill steak for 4-5 minutes per side.
    - Top with butter before serving.

2. Keto-Carnivore Meal Plan

Incorporates some low-carb, animal-based ingredients for those transitioning from a ketogenic diet or needing slight dietary flexibility.

Day 1

- **Breakfast: Bacon and Avocado**
  Ingredients:
    - 4 slices of bacon

- ○ 1 avocado
- ○ Salt to taste

Instructions:

- ○ Cook bacon in a skillet until crispy.
- ○ Slice the avocado and season with salt.
- ○ Serve bacon with avocado on the side.

- **Lunch: Ground Beef with Butter and Cheese**

Ingredients:

- ○ 1 lb ground beef (80/20)
- ○ 2 tbsp butter
- ○ 1 oz cheddar cheese

Instructions:

- ○ Cook ground beef in a skillet over medium heat.
- ○ Add butter and melt into the beef.
- ○ Top with shredded cheddar cheese.

- **Dinner: Grilled Ribeye with Ghee**

Ingredients:

- ○ 1 ribeye steak (10 oz)

- 2 tbsp ghee

Instructions:

- Grill ribeye steak to desired doneness (4-5 minutes per side for medium).
- Drizzle with ghee before serving.

Day 2

- **Breakfast: Scrambled Eggs with Bacon Fat**

Ingredients:

- 3 eggs
- 1 tbsp bacon fat
- Salt to taste

Instructions:

- Heat bacon fat in a skillet.
- Scramble eggs and cook until set.

- **Lunch: Pork Belly with Guacamole**

Ingredients:

- 6 oz pork belly

- o 1/2 avocado
- o Salt and lime juice to taste

Instructions:

- o Sear pork belly strips in a skillet until crispy.
- o Mash avocado with lime juice and salt for guacamole.
- o Serve pork belly with guacamole.

- **Dinner: Salmon with Spinach and Butter**

Ingredients:

- o 6 oz salmon fillet
- o 1 cup spinach
- o 2 tbsp butter

Instructions:

- o Pan-sear salmon for 4-5 minutes per side.
- o Sauté spinach in butter until wilted.
- o Serve salmon with spinach.

Day 3

- **Breakfast: Egg and Cheese Muffins**

  Ingredients:

  - 3 eggs

  - 1 oz cheese (cheddar or mozzarella)

  - 1 tbsp butter

  Instructions:

  - Preheat oven to 350°F (175°C).

  - Beat eggs and mix with shredded cheese.

  - Pour mixture into muffin tins and bake for 12-15 minutes.

- **Lunch: Grilled Chicken Thighs with Olive Oil**

  Ingredients:

  - 4 chicken thighs

  - 2 tbsp olive oil

  - Salt to taste

  Instructions:

- o Preheat grill to medium-high heat.
- o Rub chicken thighs with olive oil and salt.
- o Grill for 6-7 minutes per side until cooked through.

- **Dinner: Lamb Chops with Herb Butter**

Ingredients:

- o 2 lamb chops
- o 2 tbsp herb-infused butter

Instructions:

- o Sear lamb chops in a skillet over medium-high heat for 4-5 minutes per side.
- o Top with herb butter before serving.

Day 4

- **Breakfast: Sausage and Eggs**

Ingredients:

- 2 sausage links (sugar-free)
- 3 eggs
- Salt to taste

Instructions:

- Cook sausages in a skillet until browned.
- Scramble eggs in the same skillet with sausage drippings.

- **Lunch: Beef Liver with Ghee**

Ingredients:

- 6 oz beef liver
- 2 tbsp ghee
- Salt to taste

Instructions:

- Sauté liver in ghee for 2-3 minutes per side.
- Season with salt and serve.

- **Dinner: Grilled Shrimp with Zucchini**

Ingredients:

- 8 oz shrimp

- o 1 zucchini
- o 2 tbsp butter

Instructions:

- o Grill shrimp for 2-3 minutes per side.
- o Slice zucchini and sauté in butter until tender.
- o Serve shrimp with sautéed zucchini.

Day 5

- **Breakfast: Bacon-Wrapped Eggs**

Ingredients:

- o 2 eggs
- o 2 slices of bacon

Instructions:

- o Wrap each egg with a slice of bacon.
- o Bake at 375°F (190°C) for 10-12 minutes until eggs are set.

- **Lunch: Beef Stew with Bone Broth**

Ingredients:

  - 8 oz beef stew meat
  - 2 cups bone broth
  - 1 tbsp butter

  Instructions:

  - Brown beef stew meat in butter in a pot.
  - Add bone broth and simmer for 45 minutes until beef is tender.

- **Dinner: Grilled Tuna Steaks**

Ingredients:

  - 2 tuna steaks (6 oz each)
  - 1 tbsp olive oil

  Instructions:

  - Brush tuna steaks with olive oil and season with salt.
  - Grill for 3-4 minutes per side for medium-rare.

Day 6

- **Breakfast: Steak and Eggs**

  Ingredients:

  - 6 oz steak (your choice)
  - 2 eggs
  - 1 tbsp butter

  Instructions:

  - Grill or pan-sear steak to desired doneness.
  - Fry eggs in butter and serve alongside steak.

- **Lunch: Pork Ribs with Mustard**

  Ingredients:

  - 8 oz pork ribs
  - 1 tbsp mustard (optional)

  Instructions:

  - Grill pork ribs for 20-25 minutes, turning occasionally.

- Brush with mustard before serving (optional).
- **Dinner: Roasted Chicken with Avocado**

Ingredients:

- 1 whole chicken
- 1 avocado
- Salt to taste

Instructions:

- Preheat oven to 400°F (200°C).
- Roast chicken for 1 hour, seasoning with salt.
- Serve with sliced avocado.

Day 7

- **Breakfast: Chia Seed Pudding with Heavy Cream**

Ingredients:

- 2 tbsp chia seeds

- o 1 cup heavy cream
- o Stevia or erythritol to taste

Instructions:

- o Mix chia seeds with heavy cream and sweetener.
- o Let sit for 30 minutes or overnight to thicken.

- **Lunch: Grilled Salmon with Spinach Salad**

Ingredients:

- o 6 oz grilled salmon
- o 1 cup spinach
- o 1 tbsp olive oil
- o Salt to taste

Instructions:

- o Grill salmon for 4-5 minutes per side.
- o Toss spinach with olive oil and salt for a salad.

- **Dinner: Ribeye Steak with Mushrooms**

Ingredients:

- o 1 ribeye steak

- o 1/2 cup mushrooms
- o 1 tbsp butter

Instructions:

- o Grill or pan-sear ribeye steak to desired doneness.
- o Sauté mushrooms in butter and serve alongside steak.

3. Flexible Carnivore Meal Plan

This plan includes a mix of carnivore foods with a bit more flexibility to include some plant-based options, ideal for those easing into the carnivore diet or preferring some diversity.

Day 1

- **Breakfast: Scrambled Eggs with Spinach and Bacon**
  Ingredients:

- o 3 eggs
- o 1/2 cup spinach
- o 2 slices of bacon

Instructions:

- o Cook bacon until crispy, then set aside.
- o Sauté spinach in the same skillet.
- o Scramble eggs and combine with spinach and bacon.

- **Lunch: Chicken Salad with Avocado**

Ingredients:

- o 1 grilled chicken breast
- o 1/2 avocado
- o 1 tbsp olive oil

Instructions:

- o Dice chicken breast and avocado.
- o Toss with olive oil and season with salt.

- **Dinner: Beef Stir-Fry with Vegetables**

Ingredients:

- o 6 oz beef strips

- o 1/2 cup bell peppers
- o 1/4 cup onions
- o 1 tbsp soy sauce

Instructions:

- o Stir-fry beef strips in olive oil until browned.
- o Add bell peppers, onions, and soy sauce, cooking for 5 minutes.

Day 2

Breakfast: Scrambled Eggs with Bacon
Ingredients:

- 3 eggs
- 3 slices of bacon
- 1 tbsp butter

Instructions:

- Cook the bacon in a skillet until crispy, then set aside.

- In the same skillet, melt butter and scramble the eggs until cooked to your liking.
- Serve scrambled eggs with crispy bacon.

Lunch: Ground Beef and Avocado Salad

Ingredients:

- 6 oz ground beef
- 1 avocado, diced
- 1 cup mixed greens (spinach, arugula, etc.)
- 1 tbsp olive oil
- Salt and pepper to taste

Instructions:

- Cook ground beef in a skillet until browned, then season with salt and pepper.
- Toss mixed greens, avocado, and olive oil together.
- Top the salad with the cooked ground beef and serve.

Dinner: Grilled Salmon with Asparagus

Ingredients:

- 1 salmon fillet (6 oz)
- 1 cup asparagus spears
- 1 tbsp olive oil
- Salt and pepper to taste

Instructions:

- Preheat the grill or a grill pan to medium-high heat.
- Drizzle salmon and asparagus with olive oil, then season with salt and pepper.
- Grill the salmon for 4-5 minutes per side and the asparagus for about 5-7 minutes until tender.
- Serve grilled salmon with asparagus.

Day 3

Breakfast: Steak and Eggs

Ingredients:

- 1 steak (6 oz)
- 2 eggs
- 1 tbsp butter

Instructions:

- Cook the steak in a skillet over medium-high heat to your desired doneness.
- In the same skillet, melt butter and fry eggs.
- Serve the steak with eggs on the side.

Lunch: Chicken Salad with Bacon

Ingredients:

- 2 cooked chicken breasts (shredded)
- 3 slices of bacon (cooked and crumbled)
- 1/4 cup mayonnaise
- 1 tbsp mustard
- Salt and pepper to taste

Instructions:

- Shred the cooked chicken breasts and place in a bowl.
- Add mayonnaise, mustard, crumbled bacon, salt, and pepper, then mix until well combined.
- Serve chilled or at room temperature.

Dinner: Beef Liver and Spinach Sauté

Ingredients:

- 4 oz beef liver
- 1 cup spinach
- 1 tbsp butter
- Salt and pepper to taste

Instructions:

- Sauté beef liver in butter until cooked through, about 4-5 minutes per side.
- Remove liver from the pan and add spinach, cooking until wilted.
- Serve the liver on top of the spinach.

Day 4

Breakfast: Pork Sausages and Eggs

Ingredients:

- 2 pork sausages
- 3 eggs
- 1 tbsp butter

Instructions:

- Cook sausages in a skillet until browned and cooked through.
- In the same skillet, melt butter and scramble eggs.
- Serve sausages with scrambled eggs.

Lunch: Tuna Salad Lettuce Wraps

Ingredients:

- 1 can tuna in olive oil (drained)
- 1 tbsp mayonnaise

- 1 tsp mustard
- 2-3 large lettuce leaves (for wraps)
- Salt and pepper to taste

Instructions:

- Mix the tuna with mayonnaise, mustard, salt, and pepper.
- Spoon the tuna mixture into lettuce leaves and wrap them up.
- Serve as a fresh, low-carb lunch.

Dinner: Ribeye Steak with Roasted Broccoli

Ingredients:

- 1 ribeye steak (8 oz)
- 1 cup broccoli florets
- 1 tbsp olive oil
- Salt and pepper to taste

Instructions:

- Season the ribeye steak with salt and pepper, then cook to your desired doneness in a skillet or on the grill.

- Toss broccoli florets in olive oil, salt, and pepper, then roast at 400°F (200°C) for 20 minutes or until crispy.
- Serve steak with roasted broccoli.

Day 5

Breakfast: Avocado and Bacon Scramble

Ingredients:

- 3 eggs
- 2 slices of bacon
- 1/2 avocado, diced
- 1 tbsp butter

Instructions:

- Cook bacon until crispy, then crumble it.
- In the same pan, scramble the eggs in butter.
- Add the diced avocado and crumbled bacon to the scrambled eggs and serve.

Lunch: Beef and Mushroom Stir-Fry

Ingredients:

- 6 oz ground beef
- 1/2 cup mushrooms, sliced
- 1 tbsp olive oil
- Salt and pepper to taste

Instructions:

- Heat olive oil in a skillet and sauté mushrooms until soft.
- Add ground beef and cook until browned.
- Season with salt and pepper, then serve.

Dinner: Grilled Shrimp with Zucchini Noodles

Ingredients:

- 6 oz shrimp, peeled and deveined
- 1 zucchini, spiralized
- 1 tbsp olive oil
- Salt and pepper to taste

Instructions:

- Grill shrimp for 2-3 minutes per side until cooked through.
- Sauté zucchini noodles in olive oil for 3-4 minutes until tender.
- Serve grilled shrimp on top of zucchini noodles.

Day 6

Breakfast: Egg Muffins with Bacon
Ingredients:

- 3 eggs
- 2 slices of bacon
- 1/4 cup shredded cheese (optional)
- Salt and pepper to taste

Instructions:

- Preheat the oven to 375°F (190°C).
- Whisk eggs, then pour into muffin tin.

- Cook bacon and crumble it into the eggs, adding cheese if desired.
- Bake for 12-15 minutes until eggs are set.

Lunch: Salmon Salad with Avocado

Ingredients:

- 1 can of salmon (or fresh cooked salmon)
- 1/2 avocado, sliced
- 1 cup mixed greens
- 1 tbsp olive oil
- Salt and pepper to taste

Instructions:

- Flake the salmon and toss with mixed greens, avocado, olive oil, salt, and pepper.
- Serve as a light and refreshing lunch.

Dinner: Pork Belly with Cabbage

Ingredients:

- 6 oz pork belly
- 1/2 cup cabbage, shredded

- 1 tbsp butter
- Salt and pepper to taste

Instructions:

- Sear the pork belly in a skillet until crispy.
- In the same pan, sauté shredded cabbage in butter until tender.
- Serve pork belly on top of sautéed cabbage.

Day 7

Breakfast: Beef Sausages with Scrambled Eggs
Ingredients:

- 2 beef sausages (sugar-free)
- 3 eggs
- 1 tbsp butter

Instructions:

- Cook sausages in a skillet until browned and cooked through.

- In the same skillet, melt butter and scramble eggs until cooked to your liking.
- Serve sausages with scrambled eggs.

Lunch: Grilled Chicken Thighs with Mixed Greens
Ingredients:

- 2 chicken thighs
- 1 cup mixed greens (spinach, arugula, kale, etc.)
- 1 tbsp olive oil
- Salt and pepper to taste

Instructions:

- Grill chicken thighs for 6-7 minutes per side until fully cooked.
- Toss mixed greens with olive oil, salt, and pepper.
- Serve grilled chicken on top of the salad.

Dinner: Pork Chops with Roasted Brussels Sprouts

Ingredients:

- 2 pork chops (6 oz each)
- 1 cup Brussels sprouts, halved
- 2 tbsp olive oil
- Salt and pepper to taste

Instructions:

- Preheat oven to 400°F (200°C).
- Rub pork chops with olive oil, salt, and pepper, then pan-sear on both sides until golden brown.
- Transfer to the oven and roast for 10-12 minutes until cooked through.
- Toss Brussels sprouts in olive oil, salt, and pepper, and roast on a baking sheet for 20-25 minutes, stirring halfway through.
- Serve pork chops with roasted Brussels sprouts.

Day 7

- **Breakfast: Beef Sausages with Scrambled Eggs**
  Ingredients:
    - 2 beef sausages (sugar-free)
    - 3 eggs
    - 1 tbsp butter

  Instructions:
    - Cook sausages in a skillet until browned and cooked through.
    - In the same skillet, melt butter and scramble eggs until cooked to your liking.
    - Serve sausages with scrambled eggs.

- **Lunch: Grilled Chicken Thighs with Mixed Greens**
  Ingredients:
    - 2 chicken thighs

- 1 cup mixed greens (spinach, arugula, kale, etc.)
- 1 tbsp olive oil
- Salt and pepper to taste

Instructions:

- Grill chicken thighs for 6-7 minutes per side until fully cooked.
- Toss mixed greens with olive oil, salt, and pepper.
- Serve grilled chicken on top of the salad.

- **Dinner: Pork Chops with Roasted Brussels Sprouts**

Ingredients:

- 2 pork chops (6 oz each)
- 1 cup Brussels sprouts, halved
- 2 tbsp olive oil
- Salt and pepper to taste

Instructions:

- Preheat the oven to 400°F (200°C).

- o Rub pork chops with olive oil, salt, and pepper, then pan-sear on both sides until golden brown.
- o Transfer to the oven and roast for 10-12 minutes until cooked through.
- o Toss Brussels sprouts in olive oil, salt, and pepper, and roast on a baking sheet for 20-25 minutes, stirring halfway through.
- o Serve pork chops with roasted Brussels sprouts.

Quick and Easy Recipes for Busy Days

Life can get hectic, but sticking to your carnivore diet doesn't have to be complicated. These quick recipes are perfect for busy schedules without compromising flavor or nutrition.

1. 5-Minute Ground Beef Bowl

- **Ingredients:**
    1. 1 lb ground beef
    2. Salt and pepper to taste
    3. Optional: shredded cheese or a dollop of sour cream
- **Instructions:**
    1. Heat a skillet over medium heat.
    2. Cook the ground beef, breaking it up with a spatula.
    3. Season with salt and pepper. Serve immediately.

2. Air-Fried Chicken Wings

- **Ingredients:**
    1. 10 chicken wings
    2. 1 tbsp salt
    3. 1 tsp paprika
- **Instructions:**
    1. Season the chicken wings with salt and paprika.
    2. Place them in an air fryer and cook at 400°F for 20 minutes, flipping halfway through.

3. Steak in Butter Sauce

- **Ingredients:**
    1. 1 ribeye steak
    2. 2 tbsp butter
    3. 1 clove garlic, minced
- **Instructions:**

1. Sear the steak in a hot skillet for 3-4 minutes on each side.
2. Add butter and garlic to the skillet, basting the steak as it cooks.
3. Remove from heat and let rest for 5 minutes before serving.

4. Carnivore Breakfast Muffins

- **Ingredients:**
  1. 6 eggs
  2. 1/2 cup diced bacon
  3. 1/4 cup shredded cheese (optional)
- **Instructions:**
  1. Preheat oven to 375°F.
  2. Whisk eggs and mix in bacon and cheese.
  3. Pour into a greased muffin tin and bake for 15-20 minutes.

Advanced Cooking Techniques for Meat Lovers

For those who want to take their carnivore cooking to the next level, mastering these techniques will enhance the flavor and texture of your meals.

1. Dry-Aging Beef at Home

- **What You'll Need:** A mini-fridge, a wire rack, and cheesecloth.
- **Steps:**
    1. Wrap a large cut of beef (e.g., ribeye roast) in cheesecloth.
    2. Place it on a wire rack in the fridge for 7-30 days.
    3. Trim off the outer layer before cooking.

Result: Intensely flavored, tender beef that rivals restaurant-quality steaks.

2. Sous Vide Perfection

- **Why Use It:** Sous vide ensures precise temperature control for perfectly cooked meat.
- **How To:**
  1. Season your meat and vacuum-seal it in a bag.
  2. Submerge it in a sous vide water bath at your desired temperature.
  3. Finish with a quick sear in a hot skillet.

Example: Cook a ribeye at 129°F for medium-rare, then sear for 30 seconds per side.

3. Smoking Meats for Flavor

- **Essential Equipment:** A smoker or grill with wood chips.
- **Steps:**
  1. Preheat the smoker to 225°F.
  2. Season the meat with salt and spices.
  3. Smoke until the internal temperature reaches your preference (e.g., brisket at 203°F).

Tip: Experiment with different wood types like hickory, mesquite, or applewood for unique flavors.

4. Perfecting Organ Meats

Organ meats can be intimidating, but proper preparation makes them delicious.

Liver Pâté Recipe:

- **Ingredients:**

1. 1 lb chicken livers
2. 1/2 cup butter
3. 1 small onion, diced

- **Instructions:**

  1. Sauté onions in butter until soft.
  2. Add chicken livers and cook until no longer pink.
  3. Blend the mixture until smooth and chill before serving.

Supplements, Hydration, and Electrolytes

When following a carnivore diet, your body undergoes a significant shift in how it processes and utilizes nutrients. While the primary focus is on animal-based foods, it's essential to understand how to support your body's nutritional needs beyond what is provided by meat alone. Supplements, hydration, and electrolyte balance play a crucial role in ensuring that you remain healthy and energized as you adapt to this high-protein, zero-carb lifestyle. This chapter will explore whether you need supplements on the carnivore diet, the importance of staying hydrated, and how to balance electrolytes to maintain optimal performance.

Do You Need Supplements on Carnivore?

One of the most common questions for those starting the carnivore diet is whether supplements are necessary. The idea of eating only meat and eliminating plant-based foods can make some people worry about potential nutrient deficiencies. After all, plants are a rich source of vitamins and minerals, so can a meat-only diet provide everything you need?

The answer depends on various factors, including your individual health needs, the quality of the meat you consume, and how strictly you follow the carnivore diet. Let's break down some of the key nutrients and whether you may need supplements.

Key Nutrients and Potential Deficiencies

- **Vitamin C**: One of the most commonly discussed concerns is vitamin C, which is typically found in fruits and vegetables. However, the carnivore diet doesn't inherently lack vitamin C. While it's true that meat contains very little vitamin C, research has shown that a well-balanced carnivore diet can support healthy levels of vitamin C through a process called "metabolic adaptation." This means that your body can reduce the need for vitamin C when consuming a meat-based diet. Furthermore, organ meats like liver contain small amounts of vitamin C, which can help bridge the gap.

- **Vitamin D**: Vitamin D is another nutrient that people worry about when eliminating plant-based foods. Meat, especially fatty fish and organ meats, can provide vitamin D, but many people find it difficult to meet their needs through diet alone, especially if they live in areas with limited sunlight. In such cases, supplementation with vitamin D may be beneficial, particularly during the winter months when sun exposure is minimal.

- **Magnesium**: Magnesium is a mineral that plays a crucial role in muscle function, nerve transmission, and energy production. While animal products like beef, pork, and organ meats do contain magnesium, it may not be enough for some individuals. If you're feeling muscle cramps or fatigue, magnesium supplementation might be necessary to restore balance, especially during the initial stages of the carnivore diet when your body is adjusting to a low-carb state.

- **Omega-3 Fatty Acids**: Omega-3s are essential fatty acids that support heart health, brain function, and inflammation control. While grass-fed meat contains more omega-3s than grain-fed meat, the overall omega-3 content in a carnivore diet may be lower than what's found in a traditional diet with fish and plant-based sources like flaxseeds. If you're not consuming fatty fish like salmon or sardines regularly, you might want to consider supplementing with a high-quality fish oil or algae-based omega-3 supplement.

- **Iodine**: Iodine is an essential nutrient that supports thyroid function, and it's often found in sea vegetables, dairy, and iodized salt. On a carnivore diet, iodine may be limited, particularly if you're not eating seafood regularly. While iodine deficiency is rare, those who follow a strict carnivore diet may want to consider an iodine supplement or increase their intake of seafood, which is a rich source of this nutrient.

When to Consider Supplements

In general, a well-balanced carnivore diet rich in a variety of animal products, including meat, organ meats, eggs, and fish, should provide most of the nutrients your body needs. However, if you're noticing signs of fatigue, muscle cramps, or other symptoms of deficiency, it might be worth considering a supplement. It's always a good idea to consult with a healthcare provider or a nutritionist to assess your individual needs.

Staying Hydrated and Balancing Electrolytes

One of the biggest adjustments to the carnivore diet is the shift from a carbohydrate-based fuel system to a fat-based one. This change can have a profound effect on your hydration levels and electrolyte balance. Understanding how to stay hydrated and maintain your electrolytes is crucial for avoiding common pitfalls such as dehydration, fatigue, and muscle cramps.

Why Hydration Is Important on Carnivore

The carnivore diet is inherently diuretic. When you reduce your carbohydrate intake, your body stores less glycogen, which is the storage form of glucose. For every gram of glycogen stored in your muscles, your body retains about 3-4 grams of water. Without carbohydrates, your body excretes this excess water, which can lead to frequent urination and dehydration, especially in the early stages of the diet.

Proper hydration is essential for maintaining bodily functions such as digestion, temperature regulation, and joint lubrication. On a carnivore diet, you need to be extra vigilant about drinking enough water to replenish the fluids your body is losing.

Electrolytes: The Unsung Heroes

Electrolytes are minerals that carry an electric charge and are crucial for a variety of bodily functions, including muscle contractions, nerve signaling, and fluid balance. The primary electrolytes include sodium, potassium, magnesium, and calcium. When transitioning to a carnivore diet, your body may experience an imbalance in electrolytes due to the reduction in carbohydrate intake and the increased excretion of water. Here's how you can maintain balance:

- **Sodium**: Sodium is perhaps the most important electrolyte to focus on when you're on a carnivore diet. As your body excretes more water, you also lose sodium. Since the carnivore diet typically excludes high-sodium foods like processed foods and table salt, it's important to consciously increase your sodium intake. This can be done by adding salt to your meals or drinking mineral-rich broths that contain added sodium.

- **Potassium**: Potassium helps maintain proper fluid balance and is essential for heart and muscle function. On a carnivore diet, potassium levels can drop due to the reduction in potassium-rich foods like fruits and vegetables. While meat does contain some potassium, you may need to increase your intake by consuming organ meats, which are particularly rich in potassium. If you're experiencing symptoms like muscle cramps or irregular heartbeats, it might be a sign that your potassium levels are low.

- **Magnesium**: Magnesium plays a key role in muscle function and energy production.

As mentioned earlier, magnesium may be one of the minerals you need to supplement on the carnivore diet, particularly if you're experiencing muscle cramps or fatigue. Good sources of magnesium include organ meats, fish, and bone broth. If you find it difficult to meet your magnesium needs through food alone, a magnesium supplement can be beneficial.

How to Stay Hydrated

Staying hydrated on the carnivore diet is a simple but essential part of the process. In addition to drinking plenty of water, there are a few strategies to help you stay hydrated and maintain electrolyte balance:

- **Drink Mineral-Rich Broths**: Bone broth is an excellent way to hydrate and replenish electrolytes. Not only does it provide hydration, but it also contains collagen, gelatin, and amino acids that support joint and gut health. Bone broth can be a great way to get additional sodium and potassium into your diet.

- **Electrolyte Supplements**: If you're struggling to get enough electrolytes from food alone, you can opt for an electrolyte supplement. Look for supplements that contain a balance of sodium, potassium, and magnesium, with minimal added sugars or artificial ingredients. Many athletes use electrolyte powders or tablets to help maintain hydration and balance during intense physical activity, and they can be just as beneficial on the carnivore diet.

- **Drink Water with Salt**: One of the simplest ways to replenish sodium while staying hydrated is to add a pinch of high-quality sea salt to your water. This can help restore the sodium balance in your body and reduce the risk of dehydration. It's especially helpful if you experience symptoms like dizziness, fatigue, or headaches, which can be signs of low sodium.

- **Hydrate Consistently**: Make hydration a priority throughout the day, not just when you feel thirsty. By consistently drinking water and consuming hydrating foods like bone broth, you can maintain a steady fluid balance and avoid dehydration.

The Role of Salt and Fat

Salt: A Vital Nutrient

Salt is essential on the carnivore diet, not just for flavor, but for maintaining your body's electrolyte balance. The high-protein, low-carb nature of the diet increases the excretion of sodium, so it's important to consciously add salt to your meals. Sodium helps regulate blood pressure, fluid balance, and nerve function. When you don't consume enough sodium, you may experience symptoms like fatigue, dizziness, or muscle cramps.

Fat: The Fuel of the Carnivore Diet

Fat plays a pivotal role in the carnivore diet, as it is the primary energy source. While protein is essential for muscle repair and growth, fat is the body's preferred fuel source on a low-carb diet. Consuming adequate amounts of fat ensures that you have enough energy to fuel your workouts, daily activities, and metabolic functions. Fat also helps with the absorption of fat-soluble vitamins, such as vitamin A, D, E, and K.

When it comes to fat, not all fats are created equal. Animal fats from grass-fed beef, lamb, and other high-quality meats are nutrient-dense and provide essential fatty acids that support overall health. Prioritize fats from whole animal products, such as ribeye steaks, fatty cuts of pork, and grass-fed butter, to meet your energy needs on the carnivore diet.

By understanding the importance of hydration, electrolytes, and the role of salt and fat, you can better support your body's needs as you transition to and maintain a carnivore lifestyle. With careful attention to these factors, you'll ensure that your body remains well-nourished, energized, and functioning at its best.

Part 3: Transforming Your Health

Carnivore for Weight Loss

The carnivore diet has become a popular approach for weight loss, especially among those who are tired of the endless cycle of restrictive diets that never seem to work long-term. By eliminating carbohydrates and focusing exclusively on animal-based foods, the carnivore diet taps into the body's natural fat-burning mechanisms, promoting weight loss in a way that is sustainable, straightforward, and often more effective than other methods. This chapter will explore how meat supports fat burning, how to break through weight loss plateaus, and how to manage hunger and cravings on the carnivore diet.

How Meat Supports Fat Burning

The carnivore diet focuses on animal-based foods that are rich in protein and fat, with virtually no carbohydrates. This unique approach to nutrition has several physiological effects that promote fat burning and facilitate weight loss. To understand how meat helps with fat loss, we need to examine the body's metabolic processes and how it responds to the high-protein, zero-carb nature of the carnivore diet.

The Role of Protein in Fat Loss

Protein is an essential macronutrient that plays a significant role in fat loss. It helps to preserve lean muscle mass, which is crucial for maintaining a healthy metabolism. When you consume protein, your body works harder to break it down and digest it, which results in a higher thermic effect of food (TEF) compared to fats and carbohydrates. This means that your body burns more calories simply by digesting and metabolizing protein-rich foods.

Additionally, protein helps regulate hormones related to hunger and satiety. For example, it increases levels of peptide YY (PYY) and glucagon-like peptide-1 (GLP-1), hormones that promote feelings of fullness. By increasing protein intake, you reduce the likelihood of overeating and can better manage your calorie intake without feeling deprived.

The Power of Fat for Sustained Energy

While carbohydrates are typically the body's preferred source of energy, the carnivore diet encourages the body to switch to fat as its primary fuel source. When you eliminate carbs, your body enters a state known as ketosis, where it burns stored fat for energy instead of glucose. This metabolic shift is not only effective for weight loss but also helps stabilize energy levels throughout the day.

Fat is a slow-burning fuel that provides a consistent source of energy. Unlike carbohydrates, which cause spikes and crashes in blood sugar levels, fat helps maintain steady energy, keeping hunger at bay and preventing energy slumps. When fat becomes the body's primary fuel source, you may notice fewer cravings and more stable moods throughout the day, making it easier to stick to your weight loss goals.

Fat Oxidation: Burning Stored Fat

As the body shifts from burning carbohydrates to burning fat, it starts to oxidize (break down) stored fat. This is where the magic of the carnivore diet really shines. The body's ability to tap into its fat reserves and use them for energy is enhanced by the high-fat nature of the carnivore diet. As you continue to consume more fat, the body becomes more efficient at breaking down and using stored fat for fuel.

One of the reasons why the carnivore diet is so effective for fat loss is because it maximizes the body's ability to burn fat without the need for intense calorie restriction or excessive exercise. The high fat intake keeps you satiated, so you're naturally consuming fewer calories, while the body becomes more adept at burning fat for energy.

Insulin Sensitivity and Fat Loss

Insulin is a hormone that regulates blood sugar levels and promotes fat storage. High-carb diets, especially those rich in processed foods and sugars, lead to insulin resistance, where the body becomes less responsive to insulin's signals. This results in higher levels of circulating insulin, which promotes fat storage and makes it harder to lose weight.

By eliminating carbohydrates and focusing solely on animal products, the carnivore diet reduces insulin spikes and improves insulin sensitivity. With lower insulin levels, the body is less likely to store fat and more likely to burn it for energy. This metabolic shift is a key factor in the weight loss benefits of the carnivore diet.

Breaking Through Plateaus

One of the most frustrating aspects of any weight loss journey is hitting a plateau. After experiencing rapid weight loss at the start of a new diet, many people find that their progress slows down or stalls entirely. This can happen on the carnivore diet as well, but understanding why plateaus occur and how to overcome them can help you get back on track.

Why Plateaus Happen

Plateaus are a normal part of the weight loss process, especially when following a restrictive diet like carnivore. Initially, your body may shed weight quickly due to the reduction in water retention, glycogen stores, and inflammation. However, after a period of time, your body adapts to the new eating pattern, and weight loss slows down. This adaptation is your body's way of preserving energy and ensuring that it doesn't burn through its fat stores too quickly.

Additionally, factors such as stress, sleep, and hormonal fluctuations can all play a role in causing a plateau. If you've been following the carnivore diet for a while and notice that your progress has stalled, it's essential to evaluate these factors and make adjustments where necessary.

How to Break Through Plateaus

There are several strategies you can use to break through a weight loss plateau on the carnivore diet:

- **Reassess Your Calorie Intake**: Even though the carnivore diet encourages eating until you're satisfied, some people may unintentionally eat more than they realize. While protein and fat help control hunger, it's still possible to overeat, especially if you're consuming fatty cuts of meat or snacking on high-fat foods like cheese or butter. If you've hit a plateau, try tracking your food intake for a few days to ensure that you're not consuming more calories than you need. If necessary, adjust your portions to create a calorie deficit.

- **Increase Physical Activity**: If your weight loss has slowed down, increasing your level of physical activity can help break the plateau. While the carnivore diet is not necessarily a high-intensity diet, adding in some resistance training, walking, or high-intensity interval training

(HIIT) can help stimulate fat burning and increase your metabolism.

- **Vary Your Fat Intake**: If you've been consuming mostly fatty cuts of meat, consider varying your fat intake by incorporating leaner cuts of meat or reducing the amount of added fat (e.g., butter, tallow, or oils). While fat is essential on the carnivore diet, reducing your fat intake slightly can create a more substantial calorie deficit, which may help break through a plateau.

- **Try Intermittent Fasting**: Intermittent fasting (IF) is a powerful tool that can help break through weight loss plateaus. By extending the time between meals and allowing your body to enter a fasted state, you can enhance fat burning and improve insulin sensitivity. You can start with a

12-hour fasting window and gradually increase it to 16 or 18 hours, depending on how your body responds.

- **Focus on Sleep and Stress Management**: Chronic stress and lack of sleep can sabotage your weight loss efforts, regardless of your diet. High levels of cortisol (the stress hormone) can lead to fat retention, particularly around the abdominal area. Prioritize good sleep hygiene, stress-reducing activities like meditation, and self-care practices to keep your cortisol levels in check.

- **Be Patient**: Plateaus are a normal part of the weight loss journey, and it's essential to stay patient and consistent. Remember that weight loss is not always linear, and the body may need time to adjust to your new eating habits. Stay committed to the carnivore diet, and trust the process.

Managing Hunger and Cravings

Hunger and cravings are often cited as the main reasons why people abandon their diets. The good news is that the carnivore diet is uniquely positioned to help manage both. Unlike carbohydrate-based diets that lead to blood sugar crashes and constant hunger, the carnivore diet stabilizes blood sugar and keeps you feeling fuller for longer.

The Role of Protein and Fat in Hunger Regulation

Protein and fat are two macronutrients that have been shown to promote satiety. Protein, in particular, has a high thermic effect, meaning that it takes more energy for the body to digest and metabolize. This results in a feeling of fullness that lasts longer, reducing the urge to snack between meals. Similarly, fat provides slow-burning energy, keeping you satisfied and preventing hunger pangs.

When you eliminate carbohydrates, you eliminate the blood sugar fluctuations that cause hunger. Instead of constantly battling cravings for sugary snacks, you'll find that your appetite is more stable and predictable. This is one of the reasons why many people find the carnivore diet easier to follow than other low-carb diets—it's much easier to stay full and satisfied without constantly feeling hungry.

Dealing with Emotional Cravings

Emotional cravings are another challenge that many people face, especially when transitioning to a new way of eating. These cravings are often triggered by stress, boredom, or habit, rather than genuine hunger. If you find yourself craving foods that are not part of the carnivore diet, it's essential to identify the root cause of the craving and address it.

- **Stay Busy**: Sometimes, cravings can be triggered by boredom or habit. If you find yourself reaching for food out of habit, try to keep yourself busy with an activity that distracts you, such as reading, going for a walk, or engaging in a hobby.

- **Eat More Fat**: If you're struggling with hunger or cravings, it may be a sign that you need to increase your fat intake. Fat is the most satiating macronutrient on the carnivore diet, and increasing your fat intake can help you feel fuller for longer, making it easier to resist cravings.

- **Mindful Eating**: Practicing mindful eating can also help you manage cravings. By slowing down and paying attention to your hunger cues, you can better differentiate between emotional cravings and true hunger. This can help you make more conscious decisions about what and when to eat.

The carnivore diet offers a powerful approach to weight loss, with meat serving as the cornerstone of fat burning, appetite regulation, and sustained energy. By understanding how meat supports fat loss, how to break through plateaus, and how to manage hunger and cravings, you can navigate the challenges of the diet and experience lasting results. Stay committed, be patient with yourself, and trust that the carnivore lifestyle can help you achieve your weight loss goals in a way that is both effective and sustainable.

Reversing Chronic Illness: How the Carnivore Diet Can Help Heal

Chronic illness is a growing concern in modern society, with millions of people suffering from conditions like autoimmune diseases, gut issues, and chronic pain. Many individuals with chronic conditions have tried various treatments and medications, often without finding lasting relief. The carnivore diet, which involves eliminating all plant-based foods and consuming only animal products, has gained attention for its potential to reverse or significantly improve a wide range of

167

chronic health issues. In this chapter, we'll explore how the carnivore diet can support the reversal of chronic illness, particularly in relation to autoimmune conditions, gut health, and chronic inflammation.

Carnivore and Autoimmune Conditions

Autoimmune diseases occur when the immune system mistakenly attacks the body's own cells and tissues, leading to inflammation, pain, and long-term damage. Conditions like rheumatoid arthritis, lupus, multiple sclerosis, Hashimoto's thyroiditis, and psoriasis are examples of autoimmune disorders that can severely impact quality of life. Traditional treatments often involve immunosuppressive medications and lifestyle changes, but these solutions don't always address the root causes of the disease.

The carnivore diet, with its focus on animal-based foods, has been shown to have a positive impact on autoimmune conditions. While the exact mechanisms are still being studied, there are several key ways in which the carnivore diet can support immune system regulation and help reverse autoimmune symptoms.

Eliminating Trigger Foods

Many autoimmune conditions are exacerbated by food sensitivities, particularly to certain plant-based foods. Common offenders include grains, legumes, nightshades (such as tomatoes, peppers, and eggplants), dairy, and processed foods. These foods can cause inflammation in the gut and immune system, triggering flare-ups in autoimmune conditions.

By eliminating all plant-based foods, the carnivore diet removes many of the potential triggers that contribute to autoimmune reactions. The diet is simple, consisting solely of animal products such as beef, chicken, pork, fish, and eggs, which have been shown to be less likely to provoke immune system dysregulation.

Supporting the Gut-Immune Connection

A healthy gut is crucial for a well-functioning immune system. The gut is home to a large portion of the body's immune cells, and a balanced microbiome helps regulate immune responses. In individuals with autoimmune conditions, an imbalance in gut bacteria or a compromised gut lining (often referred to as "leaky gut") can contribute to immune system dysfunction.

The carnivore diet, being free of plant-based foods that can irritate the gut, allows the digestive system to heal and reduce inflammation. Meat, particularly organ meats, is rich in nutrients that support gut health, such as zinc, collagen, and amino acids. These nutrients help repair the gut lining and promote a healthy gut barrier, which in turn supports immune function.

Additionally, by eliminating potential allergens and inflammatory compounds found in plant-based foods, the carnivore diet reduces the overall burden on the immune system, allowing it to function more effectively and potentially reduce autoimmune symptoms.

Reducing Inflammation and Immune Dysregulation

Autoimmune conditions are characterized by chronic inflammation, as the immune system mistakenly attacks healthy tissues. Inflammation is also linked to the development of many other chronic diseases, including heart disease, diabetes, and cancer. The carnivore diet has been shown to reduce systemic inflammation by removing foods that trigger inflammatory responses in the body.

Animal-based foods, particularly fatty cuts of meat, are rich in omega-3 fatty acids, which have been shown to have anti-inflammatory effects. Additionally, the absence of plant-based compounds such as lectins and phytates, which can aggravate inflammation in sensitive individuals, helps reduce overall inflammation in the body.

By providing the body with nutrient-dense foods that support the immune system and reduce inflammation, the carnivore diet can play a significant role in reversing or improving autoimmune conditions.

Healing Gut Issues with an All-Meat Diet

Gut health is a cornerstone of overall health, and many chronic illnesses can be traced back to gut dysfunction. Conditions like irritable bowel syndrome (IBS), Crohn's disease, ulcerative colitis, and general digestive discomfort are increasingly common, and they can significantly impact a person's quality of life. For those suffering from gut issues, the carnivore diet may offer a path to healing.

Gut Healing Through Elimination

The first step in healing the gut is to eliminate foods that cause irritation or contribute to gut permeability (leaky gut). The carnivore diet removes all plant-based foods, which can be difficult for some people to digest due to their fiber content, anti-nutrients, and inflammatory compounds. By eliminating these foods, the gut has a chance to rest and heal.

Meat, particularly when it's grass-fed or pasture-raised, is easily digestible and provides the body with essential nutrients that support gut healing. Collagen, found in animal connective tissue and bones, is especially beneficial for gut health. Collagen helps to repair the gut lining, reducing permeability and improving digestion.

Reducing Inflammation in the Gut

Chronic gut inflammation is a hallmark of many digestive disorders, and it can be exacerbated by plant-based foods. Foods high in fiber, such as grains and legumes, can cause bloating, gas, and discomfort in individuals with sensitive digestive systems. These foods are also high in compounds like lectins and phytates, which can irritate the gut lining and promote inflammation.

The carnivore diet, by eliminating these inflammatory foods, allows the gut to heal and reduces symptoms of gut-related conditions. The anti-inflammatory properties of animal fats and omega-3 fatty acids also help soothe gut inflammation and promote a balanced gut microbiome.

Gut Healing Through Bone Broth and Organ Meats

In addition to meat, bone broth and organ meats are two critical components of the carnivore diet that support gut healing. Bone broth is rich in gelatin, collagen, and amino acids like glycine and proline, which are essential for repairing the gut lining and promoting a healthy digestive tract. These nutrients help restore the integrity of the intestinal barrier, reducing the likelihood of leaky gut and inflammation.

Organ meats, such as liver, heart, and kidney, are incredibly nutrient-dense and provide vitamins and minerals that support digestive health. These include vitamins A, D, and K2, which play key roles in maintaining the health of the gut lining and promoting a balanced immune response.

Managing Inflammation and Chronic Pain

Chronic pain and inflammation are often intertwined, with inflammation acting as the root cause of many types of pain, including joint pain, muscle soreness, and headaches. Inflammatory conditions like arthritis, fibromyalgia, and chronic fatigue syndrome can make everyday activities difficult and painful. The carnivore diet, with its anti-inflammatory effects, offers a natural and effective way to manage chronic pain and inflammation.

The Link Between Inflammation and Chronic Pain

Inflammation is a natural response of the immune system to injury or infection, but when it becomes chronic, it can lead to tissue damage and pain. Inflammatory conditions like rheumatoid arthritis and lupus are marked by ongoing immune system activation, which causes inflammation in the joints, muscles, and other tissues. This persistent inflammation can result in pain, stiffness, and a reduced range of motion.

The carnivore diet helps reduce inflammation by eliminating plant-based foods that trigger immune responses and contribute to chronic inflammation. By focusing on animal products, which are less likely to provoke inflammation, the body can begin to repair itself and reduce pain associated with inflammatory conditions.

Omega-3 Fatty Acids and Pain Reduction

One of the most significant benefits of the carnivore diet for managing chronic pain is its high content of omega-3 fatty acids, particularly when consuming fatty cuts of meat and fish. Omega-3s are known for their anti-inflammatory properties and have been shown to reduce pain and stiffness in individuals with conditions like rheumatoid arthritis, osteoarthritis, and fibromyalgia.

Studies have demonstrated that omega-3s can help reduce the production of pro-inflammatory cytokines, which are molecules that promote inflammation in the body. By increasing omega-3 intake through animal-based foods, the carnivore diet can help lower inflammation and reduce the severity of chronic pain.

Reducing Pain Through Gut Health

Chronic gut inflammation can contribute to systemic inflammation and exacerbate pain in other parts of the body. By healing the gut through the carnivore diet, individuals may experience a reduction in inflammation throughout the body, including in areas affected by chronic pain. As the gut heals, the immune system becomes more balanced, and systemic inflammation decreases, leading to less pain and discomfort.

The carnivore diet offers a unique approach to reversing chronic illness, particularly in relation to autoimmune conditions, gut health, and chronic pain. By eliminating plant-based foods that trigger inflammation and supporting the body with nutrient-dense animal products, individuals can experience significant improvements in their health. Whether you're dealing with an autoimmune condition, chronic gut issues, or persistent pain, the carnivore diet may provide a path to healing and improved quality of life. By supporting the immune system, reducing inflammation, and promoting gut health, the carnivore diet has the potential to transform your health and help you live a pain-free, vibrant life.

Mental Health Benefits of Meat

How the Carnivore Diet Can Boost Brain Health and Well-Being

Mental health is one of the most critical aspects of overall well-being, and it's increasingly recognized that nutrition plays a vital role in shaping our mood, cognition, and emotional stability. Many people struggling with mental health issues like anxiety, depression, brain fog, and mood swings often find themselves relying on medications or other interventions that may offer temporary relief, but not lasting solutions. While the role of diet in mental health has been studied extensively, the carnivore diet is a newer approach that is gaining attention for its potential to support brain health, improve mood, and help break free from addictions to sugar and carbohydrates.

In this chapter, we will explore how the carnivore diet can benefit mental health, particularly in terms of brain function, mood regulation, and cognitive clarity. By focusing on the power of meat and animal-based products, we'll uncover the mechanisms that make the carnivore diet a powerful tool for mental well-being.

Carnivore and Brain Health:

Fueling Your Mind with Animal Products

The human brain is an incredibly complex organ, requiring a wide variety of nutrients to function optimally. The brain thrives on a combination of healthy fats, proteins, vitamins, and minerals, many of which are found abundantly in animal-based foods. On a carnivore diet, the primary fuel sources come from meat, fish, eggs, and other animal products, all of which are packed with nutrients essential for maintaining cognitive health.

The Role of Fat in Brain Function

One of the key components of the carnivore diet is its high fat content, particularly saturated fats and omega-3 fatty acids. These fats are crucial for brain health. The brain is composed of approximately 60% fat, and these fats are involved in maintaining the structure and function of brain cells (neurons). Without adequate fat intake, cognitive function can suffer, leading to symptoms such as memory problems, poor focus, and difficulty processing information.

Saturated fats, found in fatty cuts of meat, are essential for maintaining the integrity of cell membranes, which is important for communication between neurons. Omega-3 fatty acids, particularly EPA and DHA, are abundant in fatty fish and grass-fed meats, and they play a key role in reducing inflammation in the brain, improving memory, and supporting emotional stability. Studies have shown that a deficiency in omega-3s can lead to cognitive decline and an increased risk of mood disorders such as depression and anxiety.

Protein and Neurotransmitter Production

Protein is another essential nutrient for brain health. The amino acids in protein are the building blocks of neurotransmitters, the chemicals that transmit signals in the brain. Neurotransmitters such as serotonin, dopamine, and GABA are responsible for regulating mood, stress response, and cognitive function. On a carnivore diet, protein from animal products provides all the essential amino acids necessary for neurotransmitter production.

For example, tryptophan, an amino acid found in meat, is a precursor to serotonin, the "feel-good" neurotransmitter that regulates mood and emotional stability. By providing a steady supply of protein, the carnivore diet helps ensure that the brain has the necessary building blocks to produce these important chemicals, which can lead to improved mood, reduced anxiety, and better overall mental well-being.

Improving Mood, Focus, and Clarity:

How Meat Supports Mental Health

The impact of diet on mood and cognitive function is undeniable, and the carnivore diet's focus on nutrient-dense animal products can have a profound effect on mental clarity, focus, and emotional stability.

Stabilizing Blood Sugar Levels

One of the most significant benefits of the carnivore diet is its ability to stabilize blood sugar levels. High-carb diets, especially those rich in processed sugars and refined carbohydrates, can lead to blood sugar spikes and crashes, which can cause mood swings, irritability, and brain fog. On a carnivore diet, the absence of carbohydrates leads to a steady supply of energy from fat, preventing these blood sugar fluctuations and providing consistent mental clarity throughout the day.

Additionally, the carnivore diet promotes a state of ketosis, where the body uses fat as its primary fuel source instead of carbohydrates. Ketones, which are produced when the body breaks down fat, are a highly efficient source of energy for the brain. Ketones have been shown to improve focus, mental clarity, and cognitive performance, which is why many people on a carnivore diet report feeling sharper, more alert, and more productive.

Mood Stabilization and Anxiety Reduction

Many individuals with mood disorders such as depression and anxiety find relief on the carnivore diet, and one of the primary reasons for this is the diet's effect on inflammation. Chronic inflammation has been linked to the development of mental health conditions, including depression, anxiety, and cognitive decline. The carnivore diet's anti-inflammatory properties, due to its emphasis on omega-3-rich animal products and the elimination of inflammatory plant-based foods, can help reduce the underlying inflammation that contributes to these mental health issues.

Furthermore, the absence of blood sugar spikes and crashes helps to regulate mood swings. Instead of relying on quick sources of sugar for energy, the body becomes more reliant on stable fat-burning for fuel, which has a calming effect on the brain and emotions. The steady energy supply can lead to greater emotional stability, fewer mood swings, and a more balanced overall mood.

Cognitive Clarity and Mental Sharpness

The mental clarity that many people experience on the carnivore diet is often attributed to the reduction of carbohydrate intake. Carbohydrates, particularly refined sugars, can cause brain fog and reduce cognitive function, making it difficult to concentrate and think clearly. On a carnivore diet, the brain is fueled by fat and ketones, both of which provide a more stable and efficient source of energy than glucose from carbohydrates.

This mental sharpness is often reported by individuals who have transitioned to a carnivore diet, especially after the initial adaptation period. Once the body becomes fully fat-adapted, many people experience improved focus, better memory, and greater cognitive performance in their daily tasks. This is especially true for those who suffer from conditions like ADHD, where maintaining focus can be a challenge. By providing the brain with a steady supply of the right nutrients, the carnivore diet can enhance cognitive function and mental clarity.

Breaking Free from Sugar and Carb Addictions:

The Role of Meat in Reversing Cravings

Sugar and carbohydrate addiction is a pervasive issue in modern society. Many individuals find themselves caught in a cycle of cravings, constantly seeking out sugary snacks or carb-rich foods to fuel their energy levels. This cycle can lead to blood sugar imbalances, weight gain, and even mental health issues like anxiety and depression. The carnivore diet offers a solution by breaking the addiction to sugar and carbs and helping individuals regain control over their cravings.

The Addictive Nature of Sugar and Carbohydrates

Sugar and carbohydrates, particularly those found in processed foods, have been shown to have addictive properties. When consumed, they trigger the release of dopamine, a neurotransmitter associated with pleasure and reward. Over time, the brain becomes accustomed to this dopamine surge, leading to cravings for more sugar and carbs to achieve the same pleasurable response. This creates a vicious cycle where individuals feel compelled to eat more sugar and carbs, even though they know it's not beneficial for their health.

The carnivore diet helps break this cycle by eliminating all sources of sugar and carbohydrates. Without these addictive foods in the diet, the brain no longer receives the same dopamine response, and cravings begin to subside. As the body becomes adapted to burning fat for fuel instead of glucose, energy levels stabilize, and the constant desire for sugar and carbs diminishes. Over time, individuals on the carnivore diet report a significant reduction in cravings and a newfound sense of control over their eating habits.

Rebalancing Dopamine and Reducing Cravings

The carnivore diet's emphasis on protein and fat also plays a key role in balancing dopamine levels. Protein, especially from animal sources, is rich in amino acids like tyrosine, which is a precursor to dopamine. By providing the brain with the building blocks necessary to produce dopamine in a more balanced way, the carnivore diet can help regulate mood and reduce the addictive drive for sugar.

Furthermore, fat plays an important role in stabilizing blood sugar and supporting brain health. When the body is burning fat for fuel, rather than constantly relying on glucose from carbohydrates, the brain is able to function more efficiently, without the highs and lows that come with sugar consumption. This stabilization helps reduce cravings and allows individuals to break free from the cycle of sugar addiction.

The mental health benefits of the carnivore diet are vast and far-reaching. By fueling the brain with nutrient-dense animal products, the carnivore diet supports cognitive function, improves mood, reduces anxiety, and enhances mental clarity. The diet's ability to stabilize blood sugar levels, reduce inflammation, and rebalance neurotransmitters makes it an effective tool for managing mental health conditions and improving overall well-being.

For those struggling with sugar and carbohydrate addiction, the carnivore diet offers a path to freedom by eliminating the foods that trigger cravings and rebalancing the brain's dopamine response. Whether you're looking to improve your mood, sharpen your focus, or break free from the grip of sugar addiction, the carnivore diet provides a powerful solution that can transform both your mind and body.

Part 4: Addressing Controversies and Challenges

Is Meat Sustainable?

Understanding the Environmental and Ethical Implications of a Carnivore Diet

As the carnivore diet gains popularity for its potential health benefits, many individuals are asking whether it is a sustainable way of eating, both for the environment and ethically. The idea of eating only animal products raises important questions about its environmental impact, the ethics of meat consumption, and how to balance these concerns while adhering to a meat-based diet. In this chapter, we will delve into these topics to explore the sustainability of a carnivore diet, including the environmental implications of meat consumption, ethical sourcing practices, and the future of meat-based eating.

Environmental Impacts of Carnivore Eating

The environmental impact of meat consumption is a topic that has been heavily debated in recent years. Meat production, particularly from industrial farming practices, is often cited as a significant contributor to greenhouse gas emissions, deforestation, and water consumption. However, it's essential to differentiate between different types of meat production and consider the broader context of sustainable meat sourcing.

Greenhouse Gas Emissions and Climate Change

Livestock farming, especially cattle farming, has long been associated with high levels of greenhouse gas emissions, particularly methane. According to studies, cattle produce methane as part of their digestive process, and this gas is a potent contributor to global warming. Additionally, large-scale factory farming operations can produce significant amounts of carbon dioxide and nitrous oxide through the use of synthetic fertilizers, transportation, and waste management practices.

That being said, the environmental impact of meat production can vary widely depending on the type of farming practices employed. Industrial-scale meat production is generally more resource-intensive and environmentally damaging, while regenerative and sustainable farming practices aim to mitigate these impacts.

Land Use and Deforestation

Another environmental concern related to meat production is the use of land for grazing and growing animal feed. Large swaths of forests, particularly in South America, have been cleared to make room for cattle ranches and crop fields to produce feed for livestock. This deforestation not only contributes to habitat loss and biodiversity decline but also reduces the planet's capacity to absorb carbon dioxide.

However, regenerative farming practices, which focus on improving soil health and biodiversity through rotational grazing and sustainable land management, have the potential to reverse some of these negative effects. By using livestock to promote healthy grasslands and restore ecosystems, these methods can help sequester carbon in the soil and reduce the overall environmental footprint of meat production.

Water Usage

Meat production, particularly beef, is often criticized for its high water consumption. It takes a significant amount of water to raise cattle, both for drinking and for growing feed crops. However, it's important to note that water usage in meat production can vary depending on the farming methods. Regenerative and grass-fed farming methods typically use less water than conventional industrial farming practices, which rely heavily on irrigation and intensive feed crop production.

Additionally, water usage should be considered in the broader context of food production. For example, growing crops for plant-based diets also requires significant water resources, especially in areas where water is scarce. When comparing the environmental impacts of plant-based and animal-based diets, it's crucial to take a holistic approach that considers water usage, land use, and emissions across the entire food system.

Ethical Meat Sourcing

One of the key concerns with a carnivore diet is the ethics of consuming animal products. For many, the idea of eating meat raises questions about animal welfare, factory farming practices, and the moral implications of consuming animals for food. As interest in meat-based diets grows, so does the demand for ethical sourcing practices that prioritize animal well-being and responsible farming methods.

Factory Farming vs. Ethical Meat Production

Factory farming, also known as industrial farming, is often criticized for its inhumane treatment of animals, poor living conditions, and heavy reliance on antibiotics and hormones. Animals in factory farms are often kept in cramped, unsanitary conditions, leading to stress, disease, and suffering. This form of meat production is also highly resource-intensive and contributes to environmental degradation through pollution, waste runoff, and excessive resource consumption.

In contrast, ethical meat sourcing emphasizes animal welfare and responsible farming practices. This includes pasture-based systems where animals are allowed to roam freely, graze, and live in natural conditions. Grass-fed and free-range farming methods are considered more humane, as they allow animals to express natural behaviors and contribute to the restoration of ecosystems through rotational grazing and other sustainable practices.

Animal Welfare Certifications

To ensure that meat is sourced ethically, consumers can look for certifications from organizations that focus on animal welfare. Certifications such as Certified Humane, Animal Welfare Approved, and Pasture Raised indicate that the animals have been raised in conditions that meet specific standards for animal care, including access to pasture, humane handling, and minimal use of antibiotics or hormones.

In addition to these certifications, supporting local, small-scale farms that prioritize animal welfare and regenerative practices can be a powerful way to contribute to a more ethical and sustainable meat industry. By choosing to purchase meat from farms that prioritize animal well-being, consumers can help drive demand for more responsible and humane farming practices.

The Future of Meat-Based Diets

As the world becomes more conscious of the environmental and ethical implications of food production, the future of meat-based diets is likely to undergo significant changes. Innovations in sustainable farming practices, plant-based meat alternatives, and lab-grown meat are all contributing to a shift in how we think about meat consumption and its role in our diets.

Regenerative Agriculture: A Solution for Sustainable Meat Production

Regenerative agriculture is an approach to farming that seeks to restore and enhance the health of the land, improve biodiversity, and sequester carbon in the soil. This farming method involves practices such as rotational grazing, no-till farming, and the integration of livestock into crop production systems. Regenerative agriculture has the potential to reduce the environmental impact of meat production while improving the overall health of ecosystems.

By prioritizing soil health, water conservation, and biodiversity, regenerative farming can provide a more sustainable model for meat production that supports both animal welfare and environmental sustainability. Many farmers and ranchers are already adopting these practices, and as demand for ethical and sustainable meat grows, we can expect to see more widespread adoption of regenerative agriculture in the future.

Lab-Grown Meat: The Rise of Cellular Agriculture

Lab-grown meat, also known as cultured meat or cellular agriculture, is an emerging technology that aims to produce meat without the need for traditional animal farming. This process involves growing meat cells in a lab using a small sample of animal tissue, which is then cultivated into muscle tissue to create meat products.

Cultured meat has the potential to significantly reduce the environmental impact of meat production, as it requires less land, water, and energy than conventional meat farming. Additionally, it could help reduce the ethical concerns associated with traditional meat production, as no animals are harmed in the process. While lab-grown meat is still in the early stages of development and faces challenges in terms of cost and scalability, it holds promise for revolutionizing the meat industry in the future.

Plant-Based and Hybrid Meat Alternatives

Another development in the future of meat-based diets is the rise of plant-based and hybrid meat alternatives. Companies like Impossible Foods and Beyond Meat are creating plant-based products that mimic the taste, texture, and appearance of traditional meat. While these alternatives are not part of a carnivore diet, they are becoming increasingly popular as a way for individuals to reduce their environmental footprint without completely giving up meat.

Hybrid meat products, which combine plant-based ingredients with animal products, are also gaining traction. These products aim to provide a more sustainable option for consumers who want to reduce their environmental impact while still enjoying the taste and texture of meat. The future of meat-based diets may involve a combination of traditional animal products, plant-based alternatives, and lab-grown meat, offering a more sustainable and ethical approach to meat consumption.

The sustainability of a carnivore diet is a complex issue that involves considering the environmental impact of meat production, the ethics of animal welfare, and the potential for future innovations in the meat industry. While traditional meat production practices can have significant environmental and ethical implications, sustainable and regenerative farming methods, along with emerging technologies like lab-grown meat, offer promising solutions for a more sustainable future.

By choosing ethical meat sources, supporting regenerative agriculture, and staying informed about the environmental and ethical considerations of meat consumption, individuals can make choices that align with their values while still enjoying the health benefits of a carnivore diet. As the meat industry evolves, the future of meat-based diets looks increasingly promising, with the potential for a more sustainable, humane, and environmentally responsible approach to meat consumption.

Overcoming Social and Practical Challenges on a Carnivore Diet

Embarking on a carnivore diet can be life-changing, offering numerous health benefits, but it also comes with a unique set of challenges, especially when it comes to social situations and daily life. From dining out with friends to managing travel and holidays, the practical aspects of maintaining a carnivore diet require thoughtful planning, resilience, and a strong sense of commitment. In this chapter, we will explore how to navigate these challenges and stick to your carnivore lifestyle with confidence.

Dining Out on Carnivore

Dining out on a carnivore diet can feel like a daunting task, especially when you're surrounded by a variety of non-carnivore options on the menu. However, with the right approach and mindset, you can enjoy eating out without compromising your diet. It's all about making smart choices, being prepared, and communicating your needs clearly to restaurant staff.

Tips for Navigating Menus

Many restaurants offer protein-based dishes that can be adapted to fit a carnivore diet. Steaks, grilled meats, burgers (without the bun), seafood, and eggs are all common menu items that can be incorporated into a carnivore meal. When ordering, you can customize your meal by requesting that sauces, marinades, or any plant-based sides be left off the plate.

If you're unsure whether a dish aligns with your carnivore needs, don't hesitate to ask the server for more details about how the dish is prepared. For example, ask if the meat is cooked in butter (which is ideal for a carnivore diet) or whether any hidden sugars or vegetable oils are used in the preparation. Most restaurants are willing to accommodate dietary restrictions, especially if you're polite and specific about your needs.

Be Prepared with Backup Options

If you're heading to a restaurant where carnivore-friendly options are limited, it's a good idea to have a backup plan. You can carry portable, carnivore-approved snacks like jerky, boiled eggs, or a small container of cooked meat to tide you over if the menu is particularly challenging. In some cases, it may even be possible to call ahead and ask the restaurant if they can accommodate your dietary preferences.

If you're attending a social gathering or a family event at a restaurant, don't be afraid to eat before you go if the options are not suitable. This ensures that you aren't left feeling hungry or tempted by non-carnivore foods. By planning ahead, you'll feel more confident and less stressed about dining out.

Dealing with Skeptics and Critics

One of the most common challenges when following a carnivore diet is dealing with skepticism and criticism from others. Whether it's family, friends, or coworkers, not everyone will understand or support your decision to follow a meat-only diet. These reactions can range from curiosity and concern to outright criticism, which can be difficult to navigate, especially if you feel pressured to explain yourself.

Staying Calm and Confident in Your Choice

The key to dealing with critics is staying calm and confident in your decision. Understand that people may question your choices because they are unfamiliar with the carnivore diet or have preconceived notions about the health implications of eating only animal products. You don't need to engage in a lengthy debate or feel compelled to justify your choices to others. Instead, simply explain that the diet is working well for you and that you've researched it thoroughly.

It can be helpful to have a few key facts at your disposal to calmly explain the health benefits of a carnivore diet. You can mention that many people experience improvements in weight loss, mental clarity, reduced inflammation, and better digestion. If someone is genuinely curious, be open to sharing your experience, but avoid getting defensive or argumentative. Your diet is a personal choice, and as long as it's working for you, that's what matters most.

Handling Family and Social Pressure

Family gatherings or social events can be tricky, especially if you're the only one following a carnivore diet. There may be pressure to "fit in" and eat what everyone else is eating. In these situations, it's important to stand firm in your decision and politely decline foods that don't align with your diet. You can bring your own carnivore-friendly dishes to family meals or social events to ensure you have something to eat that fits your dietary needs. This can also be a great opportunity to share the benefits of the carnivore diet with others, though it's best to approach these conversations with tact and respect.

If you're attending a gathering where food is central, consider eating beforehand so you aren't tempted by non-carnivore options. This will also help you avoid feeling socially awkward if others are eating foods that don't fit your diet. If someone questions your choices, respond confidently, but don't feel the need to defend yourself unless you're comfortable doing so.

Sticking to the Diet During Holidays and Travel

Holidays and travel can be some of the most challenging times to stick to a carnivore diet, as both often involve food-centered traditions, family gatherings, and meals with friends. However, with a little planning and foresight, it's entirely possible to stay committed to your diet without feeling deprived or left out.

Holidays: Staying Strong Amid Traditions

Holidays often bring about a mix of indulgent foods, sugary treats, and traditional dishes that may not align with a carnivore diet. The key to navigating holidays successfully is to plan ahead and set clear intentions. If you're hosting a holiday meal, take charge of the menu and ensure that there are plenty of meat-based dishes available. You can still enjoy a delicious and festive meal with a variety of roasted meats, charcuterie boards, and eggs. If you're attending a family gathering, offer to bring your own carnivore-friendly dishes to share. This will ensure that you have something satisfying to eat and will also give others a chance to try something new.

For many, the temptation of holiday sweets and baked goods can be overwhelming. However, it's important to remind yourself of why you're following the carnivore diet and how it aligns with your health goals. If you find yourself in a situation where you're offered something that doesn't fit your diet, politely decline, and don't feel the need to explain yourself. Over time, friends and family will learn to respect your dietary choices, and you'll feel more empowered to stay true to your commitment.

Travel: Maintaining Your Diet on the Go

Traveling can present additional challenges when it comes to maintaining a carnivore diet. Airports, restaurants, and hotels may not always offer carnivore-friendly options, but with a little preparation, you can navigate these situations successfully.

Before you travel, plan ahead by researching nearby restaurants that offer steak, grilled meats, or seafood. If you're staying in a hotel, look for one with a kitchenette so you can cook your own meals. Packing your own meat-based snacks, such as jerky, boiled eggs, or protein bars, is another great way to ensure that you have something to eat while on the go.

When traveling by air, it's essential to bring your own food, as airport and airline food typically won't meet the requirements of a carnivore diet. A well-stocked travel cooler or insulated lunch bag with pre-packed meals will ensure you stay on track, even if options are limited during your journey.

For long trips, you may need to be creative in finding ways to get your carnivore meals on the road. If you're renting a car, stock up on portable, shelf-stable meats like jerky, canned fish, or pre-cooked meats that can easily be eaten without refrigeration. When dining out, opt for simple protein-based dishes like steaks, grilled chicken, or seafood, and ask for any sides or sauces to be omitted.

Common Pitfalls and How to Avoid Them

Adopting a carnivore diet can be an exciting and transformative experience, but like any significant lifestyle change, it comes with potential challenges. It's important to be aware of common pitfalls so you can avoid them and set yourself up for long-term success. This chapter will address some of the most common obstacles people face when transitioning to a carnivore diet, how to handle initial side effects, manage nutritional deficiencies, and ensure the sustainability of your carnivore lifestyle.

Adapting to Initial Side Effects

One of the most common challenges people face when starting a carnivore diet is the adjustment period. Since this diet eliminates all plant-based foods, your body may experience some initial side effects as it adapts to a new way of eating. These side effects are often temporary and part of the body's natural adjustment to a lower carbohydrate intake and an increase in fat and protein consumption.

The First Few Days: Keto Flu Symptoms

When transitioning from a standard mixed diet to a carnivore diet, many people experience what's known as the "keto flu," which is common among those switching to a low-carb or ketogenic diet. Symptoms of keto flu can include fatigue, headaches, dizziness, irritability, muscle cramps, and digestive discomfort. These symptoms are typically caused by a sudden reduction in carbohydrate intake, which leads to the body entering a state of ketosis. During ketosis, your body begins to burn fat for fuel instead of carbohydrates, and this shift can take a few days to a week.

How to Avoid and Alleviate Keto Flu Symptoms:

1. **Hydration**: One of the main causes of keto flu is dehydration, so it's essential to drink plenty of water. Make sure to drink at least 8 glasses of water a day, and even more if you're exercising.

2. **Electrolytes**: Along with water, your body needs an adequate supply of electrolytes—particularly sodium, potassium, and magnesium. These

minerals are essential for nerve function and muscle contraction, and low levels can exacerbate symptoms of keto flu. You can boost your electrolytes by adding extra salt to your meals or drinking electrolyte-rich bone broth.

3. **Gradual Transition**: If possible, ease into the carnivore diet by gradually reducing your carbohydrate intake over a week or two, rather than going cold turkey. This can help your body adjust more smoothly.

4. **Rest**: Give your body time to adjust. If you're feeling tired or sluggish, it's okay to rest more during the first few days. The fatigue should pass as your body adapts to burning fat for fuel.

Digestive Issues

Some people experience digestive issues when they first switch to a carnivore diet. Since the diet is free from fiber, some individuals may feel bloated or constipated. This is particularly common for those who are used to eating a high-fiber diet with lots of vegetables and grains.

How to Address Digestive Discomfort:

1. **Increase Fat Intake**: Fat is essential on the carnivore diet, not only as an energy source but also for supporting digestion. If you're experiencing digestive discomfort, make sure you're consuming enough fat. You can add more fatty cuts of meat, like ribeye steak, or incorporate healthy animal fats like butter or tallow.

2. **Bone Broth**: Drinking bone broth can be a great way to soothe digestive issues, as it

is rich in collagen, gelatin, and amino acids that promote gut health.

3. **Give It Time**: Digestive discomfort is often temporary. Your body will adapt to a lower-fiber diet over time, and many people report improvements in digestion after the first few weeks.

Understanding and Fixing Nutritional Deficiencies

While the carnivore diet is nutrient-dense and provides many essential vitamins and minerals, it's important to be mindful of potential nutritional gaps. Because the diet eliminates all plant-based foods, there are some nutrients that may be consumed in smaller amounts or not at all. Understanding these potential deficiencies and knowing how to address them will help ensure that you're meeting your nutritional needs in the long run.

Vitamin C

One of the most commonly discussed potential deficiencies on a carnivore diet is vitamin C. Since fruits and vegetables are the primary sources of vitamin C, many people worry about getting enough of this essential nutrient when eating only animal products. However, meat, especially organ meats like liver, contains small amounts of vitamin C, and most carnivore dieters report that they do not experience vitamin C deficiency.

How to Address Potential Vitamin C Deficiency:

1. **Organ Meats**: Liver and other organ meats are particularly rich in vitamin C, and they should be included regularly in your diet to help cover this need.
2. **Seafood**: Certain types of seafood, such as shellfish and fish, also contain small amounts of vitamin C.
3. **Monitor Your Health**: If you notice any symptoms of vitamin C deficiency, such as bleeding gums or easy bruising, consider incorporating more organ meats into your meals or discuss supplementation with a healthcare professional.

Magnesium

Magnesium is another nutrient that can be more challenging to obtain on a strict carnivore diet, especially since it is abundant in plant foods like leafy greens, nuts, and seeds. Magnesium is vital for muscle function, nerve health, and overall well-being.

How to Address Magnesium Deficiency:

1. **Fatty Fish**: Fish like mackerel, salmon, and sardines are good sources of magnesium, so make sure to include them in your diet.

2. **Bone Broth**: In addition to being rich in collagen, bone broth also contains magnesium, making it a great addition to your diet.

3. **Magnesium Supplements**: If you find it difficult to get enough magnesium from food sources, consider a high-quality magnesium supplement, especially if you experience symptoms like muscle cramps or sleep disturbances.

Fiber

The absence of fiber on a carnivore diet is often a concern, especially since fiber plays an important role in digestive health. While it's true that a lack of fiber can cause initial digestive discomfort, many carnivores report improved bowel regularity after the initial adaptation period.

How to Maintain Digestive Health Without Fiber:

1. **Bone Broth and Gelatin**: Collagen and gelatin in bone broth can help support digestive health, especially in the absence of fiber.

2. **Gut Healing**: The carnivore diet can promote gut healing by reducing inflammation and eliminating irritants

found in plant foods, such as lectins and oxalates. This can lead to improved digestion over time.

The Importance of Long-Term Sustainability

While the carnivore diet offers numerous benefits, it's important to approach it with a mindset of long-term sustainability. In the beginning, the diet may feel restrictive, but over time, it can become second nature. Ensuring that you can stick with it for the long haul is crucial for experiencing lasting benefits and avoiding burnout.

Avoiding Diet Fatigue

One of the main challenges of the carnivore diet is the risk of getting bored with your food choices. When you eliminate plant-based foods, you're left with a more limited range of options. However, by being creative with your meal planning, you can avoid monotony and continue to enjoy the foods you eat.

Tips for Preventing Boredom:

1. **Experiment with Different Cuts of Meat**: Don't just stick to steak and chicken. Try a variety of meats, including beef, lamb, pork, fish, and organ meats. Each has its own flavor and texture, which can keep your meals interesting.

2. **Try Different Cooking Methods**: Roasting, grilling, slow-cooking, and pan-searing are just a few ways to prepare meat. Changing up your cooking methods

can make a big difference in the flavor and texture of your meals.

3. **Add Variety with Bone Broth and Animal Fats**: Bone broth and different types of animal fats, such as butter, tallow, and lard, can add richness and variety to your meals.

Building a Support System

Having a support system in place is another key factor in the long-term sustainability of the carnivore diet. Whether it's online communities, family members, or friends who are also following the diet, having others to share your experiences and challenges with can help keep you motivated and accountable.

How to Build a Support System:

1. **Join Online Carnivore Communities**: There are many online forums and social media groups where people following the carnivore diet can connect, share tips, and provide encouragement.

2. **Involve Family and Friends**: If possible, involve your family or friends in your carnivore journey. Having a support system at home can make it easier to stay on track and share your success.

By being aware of common pitfalls and addressing potential issues like initial side effects, nutritional deficiencies, and long-term sustainability, you can set yourself up for success on the carnivore diet. With the right mindset and preparation, you'll be able to navigate these challenges and enjoy the benefits of a meat-based lifestyle for years to come.

Carnivore Diet Shopping List

Here's a detailed shopping list to set you up for success on the carnivore diet. It includes essentials, optional items, and tips to help you choose high-quality products.

Proteins: The Core of the Diet

1. **Beef (High Priority)**
   - Ribeye steaks
   - Ground beef (80/20 fat ratio preferred)
   - Beef liver (nutritional powerhouse)
   - Beef heart or kidney (optional for variety)
   - Brisket
   - Chuck roast

- o Oxtail
- o Beef bones (for bone broth)

2. **Lamb**
   - o Lamb chops
   - o Lamb shank
   - o Ground lamb
   - o Lamb liver or heart

3. **Pork**
   - o Pork chops
   - o Pork belly
   - o Bacon (uncured, sugar-free)
   - o Pork ribs
   - o Ground pork

4. **Poultry**
   - o Whole chicken (great for roasting)
   - o Chicken thighs (skin-on for extra fat)
   - o Chicken wings
   - o Duck or turkey (optional for variety)
   - o Chicken liver

5. **Seafood (Optional but Nutritious)**

- Salmon (wild-caught if possible)
- Mackerel
- Sardines (canned in water or olive oil)
- Shrimp
- Scallops
- Cod
- Tuna (fresh or canned, BPA-free cans)

6. **Other Meats**
   - Bison or buffalo
   - Venison
   - Elk
   - Goat
   - Rabbit

Fats: For Energy and Flavor

1. **Animal Fats**
   - Beef tallow
   - Pork lard

- Duck fat
- Chicken fat (schmaltz)

2. **Butter and Ghee**
   - Grass-fed butter (unsalted for cooking)
   - Ghee (clarified butter, shelf-stable)

3. **Eggs**
   - Whole eggs (pasture-raised if possible)

Optional Flavor Enhancers (Minimal Use)

1. **Herbs and Spices**
   - Salt (Himalayan pink salt or sea salt preferred)
   - Black pepper
   - Garlic powder
   - Onion powder
   - Paprika (optional)

2. **Condiments (Sugar-Free and Minimal)**

- o Mustard (check for no added sugar)
- o Hot sauce (with simple ingredients)
- o Apple cider vinegar (for marinades)

3. **Broths and Stocks**

- o Beef bone broth
- o Chicken bone broth

Supplements (If Needed)

1. **Electrolytes**

- o Magnesium citrate or glycinate
- o Potassium chloride (NoSalt or Lite Salt)
- o Sodium (additional salt intake)

2. **Optional Nutritional Supplements**

- o Cod liver oil (rich in omega-3s)
- o Collagen peptides or bone broth powder

- Vitamin D3 (if you live in low-sunlight areas)

Other Essentials

1. **Kitchen Tools**
   - Cast iron skillet or stainless steel pan
   - Slow cooker or Instant Pot (for roasts and broths)
   - Meat thermometer
   - Food storage containers (for meal prep)

2. **Pantry Staples**
   - Sardines, mackerel, or salmon (canned)
   - Freeze-dried meats (for emergencies or snacks)

Shopping Tips

- **Quality Over Quantity:** Prioritize grass-fed, pasture-raised, or wild-caught options when possible for better nutrient profiles.

- **Bulk Buying:** Purchase larger cuts of meat (like roasts) to save money and portion them at home.

- **Local Sources:** Visit farmers' markets or butcher shops for fresh, high-quality meats.

- **Label Reading:** Avoid products with added sugars, preservatives, or unnecessary ingredients.

Part 5: Living the Carnivore Lifestyle

Success Stories: Real-Life Carnivore Transformations

One of the most powerful aspects of the carnivore diet is the stories that come from people who have experienced profound changes in their health and lives by embracing an all-meat lifestyle. These success stories provide not only inspiration but also valuable insights and practical advice for those considering the diet. In this section, we'll hear from everyday individuals who made the switch to carnivore, overcame challenges, and saw remarkable transformations in both their physical and mental well-being.

Testimonials from Everyday People

Rachel: Overcoming Autoimmune Struggles

Rachel, a 35-year-old mother of two, had struggled with autoimmune conditions for years. Diagnosed with rheumatoid arthritis and Hashimoto's thyroiditis, she experienced daily pain, fatigue, and brain fog that left her feeling defeated. She had tried everything—from gluten-free to paleo diets—yet nothing provided lasting relief.

After hearing about the carnivore diet from a podcast, Rachel decided to give it a try. "At that point, I was desperate," she says. "I had nothing to lose, so I went all in on carnivore. Within a week, I noticed a significant reduction in my joint pain. My energy levels were higher, and the brain fog lifted."

For Rachel, the journey wasn't without its challenges. She initially struggled with the transition, particularly during the first few days of adjusting to the new diet. "I had cravings, and my body was used to having carbs and sugar. But I stuck with it, and within a few weeks, the cravings faded, and I started to feel better than I had in years."

Today, Rachel is pain-free, no longer dependent on medications, and has regained her energy and vitality. She continues to follow the carnivore diet and feels that it has given her a new lease on life. "I feel empowered by my diet. It has allowed me to take control of my health in a way I never thought possible."

James: Breaking Free from Obesity

James, 42, had battled obesity for most of his life. Weighing over 300 pounds and struggling with Type 2 diabetes, high blood pressure, and sleep apnea, he was stuck in a cycle of dieting, exercising, and gaining the weight back. Frustrated and desperate for a solution that would work, James came across the carnivore diet while reading about alternative approaches to weight loss. Intrigued, he decided to give it a shot.

"The first few days were rough," James admits. "I had headaches and felt tired, but I pushed through. After about a week, my energy levels started to rise, and I noticed I wasn't hungry all the time."

James' transformation wasn't just about losing weight. His Type 2 diabetes reversed, and his blood pressure returned to normal. Within a few months, he had lost 80 pounds, and his sleep apnea symptoms significantly improved. "I feel like a different person," James says. "I can play with my kids without feeling out of breath, and I've stopped taking all my medications."

James attributes his success to the simplicity of the carnivore diet. "There's no guesswork. I eat meat, and that's it. I don't have to track calories or worry about portion sizes. It's liberating."

Lily: Healing from Chronic Digestive Issues

Lily, 29, had struggled with chronic digestive issues for years. Bloating, cramps, and irregular bowel movements were constant companions, and she was often diagnosed with conditions like IBS (irritable bowel syndrome) or gluten sensitivity, though none of the treatments seemed to work. After years of trial and error with different diets, including gluten-free, paleo, and keto, she decided to give the carnivore diet a shot after seeing the testimonies of others on social media.

"The first few days were challenging—I was used to eating a lot of vegetables and fiber," Lily says. "But after a week, I noticed a huge change. My bloating started to subside, and my digestive system felt more stable. By the end of the month, I was having regular, pain-free bowel movements for the first time in years."

Now, Lily's digestion is fully healed, and she has more energy than ever before. "I don't worry about my gut anymore. I don't have to carry around medicine for bloating or cramps. The carnivore diet completely transformed my health."

Carlos: Regaining Mental Clarity and Energy

Carlos, 53, had spent years battling fatigue, poor sleep, and lack of mental clarity. As a busy executive, he often turned to caffeine and sugar to get through long workdays. Despite trying various diets and supplements to boost his energy, nothing seemed to help. When a colleague suggested trying the carnivore diet, Carlos was skeptical but willing to give it a try.

"I've always been someone who believed in balanced meals with carbs, veggies, and protein. I didn't think eating only meat would be sustainable or healthy," Carlos says. But after just a few days on the carnivore diet, he noticed a significant shift. "The brain fog started clearing, and I felt more focused. I didn't need caffeine anymore, and my energy levels were steady throughout the day."

After several months, Carlos found that his mental clarity improved drastically, and his mood was more stable. "I was sharper at work, and I felt more present with my family. The diet isn't just about weight loss—it's about mental and emotional health too."

Lessons Learned and Tips for Beginners

The success stories shared above are just a few examples of how the carnivore diet can transform lives. But these individuals didn't get to their success overnight. Along the way, they encountered challenges, learned valuable lessons, and developed strategies that helped them stay committed. Here are some key takeaways and tips for anyone starting their carnivore journey.

1. **Start Slow, Be Patient**

Many people begin their carnivore journey with high expectations. They want to feel better immediately, but the transition can take time. Whether it's adapting to a new way of eating or allowing your body to adjust to burning fat for fuel, patience is key.

James, for instance, experienced fatigue and headaches during the initial stages. "The first few days were tough, but I reminded myself that my body was adjusting. The results were worth the struggle," he says.

Start with a few days or even a week of strict carnivore eating and see how your body responds. Gradually increase the amount of meat you're eating while eliminating any lingering carb-heavy foods.

2. Prepare for Initial Challenges

The first few days or weeks on the carnivore diet can be difficult. Some common challenges include cravings, digestive discomfort, and a temporary dip in energy. However, these challenges are often short-lived as your body adjusts to its new fuel source.

Lily warns new carnivores to expect digestive adjustments. "At first, I felt bloated and uncomfortable, but that passed after a few days. It's part of the transition."

To help with the adjustment, focus on staying hydrated and getting enough electrolytes. Drink plenty of water, and consider adding salt to your meals to help with the initial side effects.

3. Be Prepared to Deal with Skeptics

When you start a carnivore diet, you may encounter skepticism and criticism from friends, family, or colleagues. Many people still view an all-meat diet as extreme or unhealthy. It's important to stay confident in your decision and remember why you chose this path.

Rachel says, "I had people telling me I was crazy, but I stuck with it because I was finally feeling better after years of suffering. Now, those same people are asking me for advice."

If you're committed to your health and well-being, stay firm in your decisions and don't let others deter you. Over time, as they see your progress, their opinions may shift.

4. Focus on the Quality of Your Meat

Choosing high-quality meat is crucial for the success of your carnivore journey. Grass-fed, pasture-raised, and wild-caught options tend to be more nutrient-dense and free from hormones and antibiotics.

Carlos learned this lesson early on: "I switched to better-quality meat, and I noticed the difference in how I felt. I had more sustained energy and less inflammation."

Prioritize quality cuts of meat that are rich in essential nutrients, such as beef, lamb, pork, and organ meats. Quality is just as important as quantity when it comes to your carnivore meals.

5. Track Your Progress

Documenting your progress is one of the best ways to stay motivated and see how far you've come. Keep track of changes in your energy, digestion, mood, and any health improvements. This not only helps you stay on course but also helps you identify what's working and what might need adjustment.

Lily suggests keeping a journal. "It helped me stay focused and see how much better I was feeling, especially when I started experiencing setbacks."

Final Thoughts:

The real-life transformations shared in these success stories illustrate the powerful potential of a carnivore diet. Whether it's reversing chronic conditions, losing weight, or enhancing mental clarity, the carnivore diet offers a simple yet effective way to improve your health and well-being. However, it's not a one-size-fits-all solution, and each person's journey will be unique. By starting slow, being patient, and learning from the experiences of others, you can set yourself up for success and achieve lasting results.

Beyond the Plate: Embracing a Carnivore Mindset

The journey to adopting a carnivore diet is more than just a change in what you eat—it's a complete shift in your mindset and how you view food, health, and wellness. As you embrace a meat-based lifestyle, you'll notice not only physical changes but also a mental transformation. It's not just about the steak on your plate; it's about how you view nourishment, discipline, and your relationship with food.

How Carnivore Changes Your Perspective on Food

When you begin a carnivore diet, you quickly realize that the focus shifts from food as a source of pleasure and indulgence to food as a source of fuel and nourishment. This shift is pivotal and often requires a mental adjustment. For many people, food has been tied to emotional fulfillment, comfort, and social bonding. The carnivore diet challenges that mindset by offering a more simplified, streamlined approach to eating—one that is grounded in the idea of optimizing health rather than satisfying cravings or indulging in variety.

The Mindset Shift: From Variety to Simplicity

Most people's diets are built around variety. We are taught to eat a balanced meal with a combination of protein, carbohydrates, fats, and a wide array of vegetables. On a carnivore diet, the concept of "variety" takes on a different meaning. It's no longer about mixing plant-based foods to create colorful meals; it's about choosing different cuts of meat, varying your protein sources, and focusing on high-quality animal products to provide the nutrition your body needs.

This simplification can feel like a breath of fresh air. The constant decision-making about what to eat, what to pair with what, and how to balance macronutrients can be overwhelming. On the carnivore diet, the decision-making is streamlined: focus on meat, and let your body tell you what works best.

The Mental Clarity of Carnivory

As you shift away from processed foods, sugars, and carbs, many people report a surprising side effect: mental clarity. A carnivore diet can help clear brain fog, improve focus, and give you a sharper sense of awareness. This is likely due to the reduction in blood sugar fluctuations and the steady supply of ketones to the brain, which is a byproduct of fat metabolism.

On a traditional mixed diet, many people experience highs and lows of energy throughout the day, often feeling sluggish after meals. With a carnivore diet, the body's constant fuel source—fat—provides steady energy. This helps you think more clearly and maintain focus throughout the day without the rollercoaster effect of insulin spikes and crashes.

Food as Fuel, Not Entertainment

On the carnivore diet, you'll find that your relationship with food changes. Meals are no longer about satisfying emotional cravings or social norms—they are about providing the body with what it needs to function at its best. Food is no longer a source of entertainment or distraction. It's fuel, and the simplicity of this approach can lead to greater appreciation for the meals you do have.

For example, rather than seeking variety in every meal, you might find that a perfectly cooked ribeye steak or a plate of grilled lamb chops provides everything your body needs. This simplicity helps eliminate the constant chatter around food and cravings that can sometimes be overwhelming on a more varied diet.

Building a Support System

Starting a carnivore diet can be a daunting experience, especially if you're making the transition alone. The mindset shift, along with the drastic changes in what you eat, can feel isolating. This is why building a support system is crucial. Having a network of like-minded individuals can provide motivation, accountability, and camaraderie, making the journey easier and more enjoyable.

Finding Like-Minded Individuals

Whether you're joining an online community, connecting with friends or family who are also following a carnivore diet, or seeking out local groups or support circles, it's essential to surround yourself with people who understand the challenges and triumphs of this lifestyle. These connections can help you stay on track when the going gets tough, offer valuable advice when you hit roadblocks, and celebrate your victories along the way.

Online forums and social media groups are excellent places to find support. Many carnivore communities on platforms like Facebook, Reddit, and Instagram provide a wealth of information, personal stories, and advice from people who have been following the diet for years. These communities can help you stay motivated and give you practical tips for navigating common challenges, such as dining out, managing social situations, or troubleshooting digestive issues.

Support From Family and Friends

Having support from your family and friends can also make a big difference. It can be difficult to stick to a restrictive diet if your loved ones aren't on board or don't understand why you're making such a drastic change. If possible, try to educate your family and friends about the benefits of a carnivore diet and share your experiences with them. You may even find that some of them are open to trying it with you or at least supporting your decision.

In some cases, you may face skepticism or concern from loved ones who don't understand the carnivore diet. It's important to be patient and provide them with information so they can understand why you're making this change. Over time, as you begin to experience the positive effects of the diet, they may become more supportive and curious about the lifestyle themselves.

Accountability Partners

One of the most effective ways to stay on track is to have an accountability partner. This can be someone you know personally or a fellow carnivore dieter you meet online. Having someone to check in with regularly, share your successes, and discuss challenges with can help keep you motivated and focused on your goals.

An accountability partner can also help you stay consistent during tough times. Whether you're experiencing cravings, social pressures, or a temporary loss of motivation, having someone to talk to can help you push through those moments and stay committed to your carnivore lifestyle.

Living a Balanced, Meat-Centered Life

Embracing a carnivore diet is about more than just eating meat; it's about adopting a balanced, holistic approach to life. While meat is the cornerstone of the diet, it's important to find balance in other areas of your life as well—your physical health, mental well-being, and social connections. By focusing on overall wellness and sustainability, you can create a fulfilling and enjoyable carnivore lifestyle.

Maintaining Physical Health

A balanced, meat-centered life involves not only nourishing your body with high-quality animal products but also incorporating physical activity, sleep, and stress management. While the carnivore diet provides the nutrients your body needs to function at its best, it's important to remember that health is multifaceted.

1. **Exercise**: Regular physical activity is crucial for overall health. Whether it's strength training, cardiovascular exercise, or simply walking, incorporating movement into your daily routine will complement the benefits of the carnivore diet and help you maintain muscle mass, improve heart health, and support mental well-being.

2. **Sleep**: Quality sleep is essential for recovery and well-being. Prioritize sleep by establishing a consistent bedtime routine and creating a restful sleep environment. Sleep plays a vital role in

regulating hormones, improving mood, and supporting cognitive function.

3. **Stress Management**: Chronic stress can negatively impact your health, so it's important to manage stress through techniques such as mindfulness, meditation, deep breathing, or spending time in nature. Stress management supports your mental and physical health, helping you stay resilient on your carnivore journey.

Social and Cultural Balance

Living a carnivore lifestyle doesn't mean isolating yourself from social events or cultural experiences. While it can be challenging to navigate social gatherings, dining out, or holidays on a carnivore diet, with the right mindset and preparation, it's entirely possible to enjoy these experiences without feeling deprived or alienated.

For example, when dining out, many restaurants now offer protein-heavy dishes like steaks, grilled fish, and rotisserie chicken. You can ask for modifications, such as swapping out the starches for extra meat or a side of salad (if you follow a more flexible version of carnivory). By being prepared and confident in your dietary choices, you can enjoy meals out without stress or guilt.

During holidays and family gatherings, focus on the social aspects of the occasion rather than the food. You can bring your own carnivore-friendly dishes to share, ensuring that you have options available. Over time, friends and family will come to respect your choices and may even begin to embrace them themselves.

Sustainability and Enjoyment

Sustainability is key to long-term success on the carnivore diet. By building a balanced lifestyle that includes variety in your food choices, regular exercise, good sleep, and social connections, you can create a sustainable carnivore life that supports both your health and happiness.

The carnivore diet is not just about food; it's about adopting a new way of living that prioritizes simplicity, nourishment, and well-being. By embracing the carnivore mindset, building a supportive community, and finding balance in all areas of life, you can make the carnivore diet a sustainable and rewarding lifestyle.

Your Carnivore Cure Blueprint

The carnivore diet has the potential to transform your health in ways you may not have thought possible. However, as with any significant lifestyle change, the key to success lies in creating a personalized plan that suits your needs, goals, and unique circumstances. This blueprint is your final guide to turning everything you've learned from this book into actionable steps to help you succeed on your carnivore journey.

In this section, we will break down key takeaways from the book, guide you in creating your own personalized carnivore plan, and help you move forward with confidence.

Key Takeaways from the Book

The carnivore diet is not a "one-size-fits-all" solution, but rather a tailored approach to eating that emphasizes simplicity, nutritional density, and healing power. Let's review some of the most crucial insights from the book:

1. The Power of Meat-Based Nutrition

By focusing on animal-based foods, the carnivore diet provides your body with the most bioavailable nutrients, especially protein and fats. These macronutrients are essential for everything from muscle repair to hormone production and immune function. The lack of carbs in the diet forces your body to burn fat for fuel, which has profound implications for weight loss and energy levels.

2. Healing Chronic Conditions

The carnivore diet has proven effective in reducing symptoms of autoimmune diseases, chronic inflammation, and gut issues. Whether it's healing the gut, reducing autoimmune flare-ups, or alleviating chronic pain, eliminating plant-based foods can help give your body the clean slate it needs to repair itself.

3. Mental Health Boost

Many people experience improvements in mental clarity, mood, and energy when transitioning to a meat-based diet. The diet's focus on nutrient-dense foods like organ meats and fatty cuts of meat provides the brain with essential nutrients that promote cognitive function, emotional stability, and focus.

4. Sustainability Through Simplicity

One of the greatest advantages of the carnivore diet is its simplicity. Unlike other diets that require complex meal planning or constant calorie tracking, the carnivore diet allows you to focus on high-quality meats, simplifying your meals and eliminating unnecessary food stress.

5. The Carnivore Diet Is Not a Quick-Fix

While the benefits of the carnivore diet are profound, it's essential to recognize that transformation takes time. Your body will go through an adjustment period, and the healing process can be gradual. The initial phase might be challenging, but staying committed will reward you with long-term, sustainable health benefits.

Creating Your Personalized Plan

As you embark on the carnivore journey, creating a plan that aligns with your goals and lifestyle is crucial. Here's how to approach it:

1. Set Clear Goals

Before diving into the diet, take a moment to reflect on your motivations. Are you seeking to lose weight, alleviate chronic health issues, or improve mental clarity? Setting clear and realistic goals will keep you focused and help you track your progress.

For example:

- **Weight Loss**: If your primary goal is weight loss, focus on consuming fatty cuts of meat to stay satiated, while gradually reducing your caloric intake.

- **Healing Chronic Illness**: If you're following the diet to manage conditions like autoimmune diseases, it might take a few weeks or months to notice significant improvements, so be patient.

- **Mental Clarity**: For those seeking cognitive enhancement, including organ meats like liver can provide essential nutrients for brain health.

2. Start with a Clean Slate

The transition to carnivore is best achieved by starting with a clean slate. This means eliminating all plant-based foods, processed foods, and sugars from your diet. You'll want to completely cut out carbs to allow your body to begin using fat for energy.

Pantry Purge: Begin by going through your kitchen and removing any non-carnivore foods. This includes grains, fruits, vegetables, and processed foods. Stock up on high-quality meats, including beef, lamb, pork, and organ meats.

Transitioning Gradually: If you've been eating a standard mixed diet, consider transitioning gradually. Start by cutting out processed foods and focusing on animal-based meals. Over time, reduce your carb intake until you're fully on the carnivore path.

3. Choose Your Meats Wisely

Quality matters when it comes to your meat-based meals. Opt for grass-fed, pasture-raised, and wild-caught options when possible. These meats are richer in omega-3 fatty acids and other essential nutrients. When selecting cuts of meat, prioritize fatty cuts like ribeye steaks, pork belly, and ground beef with a higher fat content.

Don't forget the importance of organ meats, such as liver, heart, and kidneys, which are packed with vitamins and minerals that are hard to find in muscle meat alone. Bone broth is another excellent source of nutrients and can help support joint health, gut healing, and overall recovery.

4. Listen to Your Body

Your body will give you feedback during this transition period. Pay attention to how you feel—whether that's more energy, fewer cravings, or even detox symptoms like headaches or fatigue. This is normal during the early stages of the diet as your body adjusts.

Some people may experience constipation or digestive issues in the first week of carnivore. Make sure to stay hydrated, and if needed, add extra electrolytes through salt and water. After your body adapts to fat-burning, these issues will usually resolve.

5. Stay Hydrated and Balance Electrolytes

Proper hydration is essential, as you may experience increased water loss during the early phase of the carnivore diet. It's important to drink plenty of water throughout the day and ensure that your electrolytes are in balance.

Consider adding salt to your meals to maintain sodium levels, and supplement with magnesium and potassium if needed. These adjustments will help reduce the common symptoms of fatigue, muscle cramps, and dizziness that sometimes occur during the diet transition.

6. **Plan for Challenges**

No diet is without its challenges, and the carnivore diet is no exception. Whether you're dealing with cravings, social situations, or a lack of variety, it's crucial to have strategies in place to overcome obstacles.

- **Social Situations**: When dining out, focus on ordering simple dishes that emphasize meat—grilled steaks, burgers without buns, or roasted chicken. Most restaurants are willing to accommodate your dietary preferences.

- **Cravings**: If cravings strike, remember that they are temporary. The more you stick to the diet, the fewer cravings you'll experience. Keep your meals satisfying by prioritizing fatty cuts of meat, which help keep you full longer.

7. Track Your Progress

It's essential to track your progress as you transition to carnivore. Keep a journal to monitor changes in your health, energy levels, mental clarity, and any other key markers you're focusing on. This will not only help you see how far you've come but also give you insight into how your body is responding to different aspects of the diet.

Some key metrics to track include:

- Weight and body composition (if weight loss is a goal)
- Sleep quality
- Energy levels throughout the day

- Mood and mental clarity

By tracking your progress, you can make adjustments to your diet and lifestyle as needed.

Moving Forward with Confidence

The final step in your carnivore journey is moving forward with confidence. This diet isn't just about eating meat; it's about embracing a mindset of health and vitality. You've learned how to make the diet work for you, and now it's time to fully integrate it into your lifestyle.

1. Embrace the Long-Term Commitment

The carnivore diet is not a quick-fix solution but a lifestyle choice that can deliver long-lasting health benefits. As you continue on this path, embrace the long-term commitment. This diet will help you break free from the cycle of dieting, cravings, and reliance on processed foods.

2. Stay Consistent and Be Patient

Consistency is key when it comes to any diet, and the carnivore lifestyle is no different. Be patient with your body as it adjusts, and stay consistent in your efforts. As you continue with the diet, you'll experience even greater benefits over time.

3. Share Your Success

Once you start to experience the benefits of the carnivore diet, share your success with others. You may become a source of inspiration and motivation for those around you who are struggling with their own health issues. Whether through social media, support groups, or just word of mouth, your transformation could help someone else find the path to better health.

In conclusion, the carnivore diet offers a transformative path to health, but it requires careful planning, patience, and commitment. By following the personalized blueprint you've crafted, you can enjoy the benefits of a meat-based lifestyle—whether it's weight loss, healing from chronic conditions, or boosting mental clarity. Embrace the process, stay focused on your goals, and move forward with confidence, knowing that this diet has the power to change your life.

Conclusion

The carnivore diet has been more than just a change in how I eat—it's been a complete transformation of how I view health, food, and even life itself. What started as a personal experiment to heal my body and mind turned into a journey of discovery, growth, and empowerment. I've experienced firsthand the profound benefits of this way of eating, and I've seen how it has changed the lives of so many others.

In this conclusion, I want to share why I believe the "Carnivore Cure" is truly worth it and my vision for a future where more people embrace the power of a meat-based diet—not just for their health, but for a more sustainable and balanced way of living.

Final Thoughts: Why the Carnivore Cure Is Worth It

Healing That Feels Like Freedom

When I first started the carnivore diet, I had no idea how much it would change my life. I was tired of feeling stuck—physically, mentally, and emotionally. I had tried so many diets, supplements, and strategies, but nothing gave me lasting results. The carnivore diet, however, was different.

As I eliminated processed foods, sugar, and even plants, I felt my body start to heal. My energy levels soared, my mental clarity sharpened, and chronic issues that I had struggled with for years began to fade away. It felt like my body was finally working with me, not against me.

This journey wasn't just about physical health. It was about freedom—freedom from the endless cycle of food cravings, guilt, and confusion. I stopped worrying about what to eat and started focusing on how I felt. And for the first time in years, I felt amazing.

The Beauty of Simplicity

One of the things I love most about the carnivore diet is its simplicity. I used to spend so much time planning meals, counting calories, and juggling food groups. Now, my approach to food is refreshingly straightforward: I eat high-quality meat, prepare it simply, and enjoy it without overthinking.

This simplicity has been a gift in more ways than one. It's freed up my time and mental energy, allowing me to focus on what really matters—my family, my work, and my passions. I've also found that this minimalist approach to eating has spilled over into other areas of my life. I've learned to simplify, prioritize, and let go of the unnecessary.

A Solution That Makes Sense

What makes the carnivore diet so effective is how intuitive it feels once you get started. Humans have been eating animal-based diets for thousands of years. It's only in recent history that we've moved away from this natural way of eating, and our health has suffered as a result.

For me, the carnivore diet isn't about following a trend—it's about returning to what works. It's about giving my body the most nutrient-dense, bioavailable foods possible and trusting that it knows how to heal and thrive when given the right tools.

My Vision for a Meat-Based Future

A Shift in Perspective

I believe the carnivore diet has the potential to spark a larger conversation about how we think about food, health, and sustainability. For too long, meat has been vilified in the name of trendy diets and misleading narratives. But as more people discover the healing power of meat-based nutrition, I see a future where this way of eating is embraced—not just as a diet, but as a lifestyle.

My hope is that we can move past the fear-mongering around meat and focus on the incredible benefits it provides. This isn't about pushing everyone to eat exactly like I do. It's about encouraging people to question the status quo, explore their options, and find what works best for their bodies.

Building a Supportive Community

One of the most rewarding parts of my carnivore journey has been connecting with others who are on the same path. Whether it's through online forums, social media, or casual conversations, I've been inspired by the stories of people who have transformed their lives with this diet.

My vision for the future includes a strong, supportive community of carnivore enthusiasts who can share their experiences, learn from one another, and inspire others to give this way of eating a try. No one should feel alone in their journey, and together, we can create a network of encouragement and knowledge.

A Commitment to Sustainability

I'm also deeply committed to promoting ethical and sustainable practices within the carnivore community. Choosing high-quality, responsibly sourced meat is not just better for our health—it's better for the planet. I believe that as demand for grass-fed, pasture-raised, and regenerative farming practices grows, we can create a food system that is more aligned with the values of health, sustainability, and respect for the environment.

I envision a future where meat-based diets are not only celebrated for their health benefits but also recognized as a sustainable and ethical choice. By supporting local farmers, reducing waste, and educating others about the importance of quality over quantity, we can make a positive impact on the world around us.

Moving Forward Together

As I reflect on my own journey and the incredible stories I've encountered along the way, I'm filled with hope and excitement for the future. The carnivore diet has given me so much—health, clarity, energy, and a renewed sense of purpose. And I know it can do the same for so many others.

This isn't just about eating meat; it's about reclaiming your health, your freedom, and your connection to food. It's about embracing a lifestyle that nourishes your body, respects your values, and empowers you to live your best life.

So, as you move forward, remember that you're not alone. Whether you're just starting your carnivore journey or have been living this lifestyle for years, there's a community of people who understand, support, and celebrate your choices. Together, we can challenge outdated ideas, inspire change, and create a brighter, healthier future—one bite at a time.

Let's move forward with confidence, knowing that the Carnivore Cure is more than just a diet. **It's a movement. And it's only just beginning.**

Appendices

The appendices provide additional information to support your carnivore journey. From answering common questions to offering trusted resources and scientific studies, this section is designed to equip you with everything you need to succeed and stay informed.

Frequently Asked Questions (FAQs)

General Questions

Q: Can I drink coffee or tea on the carnivore diet?

A: While the carnivore diet emphasizes animal-based foods, some people include coffee or tea, especially during the transition phase. However, for a stricter approach, eliminating all plant-based items, including beverages, is ideal.

If you choose to include coffee or tea, opt for unsweetened versions and monitor how your body reacts.

Q: Is it safe to eat only meat?

A: Yes, many people thrive on an all-meat diet. Meat provides complete proteins, essential fats, and a range of vitamins and minerals necessary for optimal health. However, it's important to include a variety of cuts and organ meats to ensure balanced nutrition.

Q: How much meat should I eat per day?

A: There's no one-size-fits-all answer. Start by eating until you're full, focusing on hunger cues rather than portion sizes. On average, many people consume 1–2 pounds of meat daily, but your needs may vary based on activity level, goals, and body size.

Q: Can I follow the carnivore diet while pregnant or breastfeeding?

A: Many women have successfully followed the carnivore diet during pregnancy and breastfeeding. Meat provides essential nutrients like iron, protein, and healthy fats, which are critical during these stages. However, consult your healthcare provider to ensure you meet all nutritional needs.

Advanced Questions

Q: What happens to gut microbiota on a carnivore diet?

A: The gut microbiome adapts to the foods you consume. On a carnivore diet, certain bacterial populations may decrease (those reliant on fiber), while others that thrive on protein and fat digestion increase. Many people report improved gut health, reduced bloating, and fewer digestive issues.

Q: Does the carnivore diet increase the risk of heart disease due to high saturated fat intake?

A: Current research challenges the traditional view that saturated fat causes heart disease. Studies show that a diet high in animal fats, when paired with low carbohydrate intake, may improve cholesterol markers, reduce inflammation, and support heart health.

Q: Is gluconeogenesis a concern on the carnivore diet?

A: Gluconeogenesis is the body's process of creating glucose from non-carbohydrate sources like protein. On a carnivore diet, this process is natural and helps maintain stable blood sugar levels. It doesn't lead to harmful glucose spikes or insulin resistance.

Q: Can I exercise while on a carnivore diet?

A: Absolutely. Many athletes and fitness enthusiasts thrive on carnivore diets, reporting improved recovery, strength, and endurance. During the adaptation phase, you might experience a temporary dip in energy, but this typically resolves as your body becomes fat-adapted.

Q: How do I handle eating out or social events?

A: Focus on simple meat-based options. At restaurants, order steaks, burgers (without buns), grilled chicken, or seafood. At social events, eat beforehand or bring your own carnivore-friendly dish. Most people are understanding if you explain your dietary choices.

Carnivore-Friendly Resources

Here are some trusted books, websites, and communities to deepen your understanding of the carnivore lifestyle and connect with like-minded individuals:

Books

1. **"The Carnivore Diet" by Shawn Baker**
   A foundational book that explores the benefits of a meat-based diet, complete with science, practical tips, and success stories.

2. **"The Carnivore Code" by Paul Saladino**
   This book delves into the ancestral and scientific basis for eating an all-meat diet,

including its impact on chronic diseases and overall health.

3. **"Sacred Cow" by Diana Rodgers and Robb Wolf**

   A comprehensive look at the nutritional, environmental, and ethical aspects of eating meat.

4. **"Ketogenic Diet" by Lyle McDonald**

   Though not exclusively carnivore-focused, this book offers insights into the metabolic effects of low-carb, high-fat diets.

Websites

1. **MeatRx (www.meatrx.com)**

   A hub for carnivore resources, including

meal plans, success stories, and a supportive community.

2. **Zeroing In On Health (www.zerocarbzen.com)**

A collection of personal stories, FAQs, and guidance for those interested in a zero-carb lifestyle.

3. **Shawn Baker's Blog (www.shawn-baker.com)**

Insightful articles, videos, and research updates from one of the leading voices in the carnivore movement.

4. **Nutrition with Judy (www.nutritionwithjudy.com)**

A wealth of resources on meat-based diets, including guides for transitioning, managing health conditions, and more.

5. **Diet Doctor (www.dietdoctor.com)**

While primarily focused on low-carb and

ketogenic diets, this site includes valuable carnivore content and meal ideas.

Communities

1. **Carnivore Cast Podcast**

   A podcast featuring interviews with experts and real-life carnivores sharing their experiences.

2. **Carnivore.Keto.Fasting Facebook Group**

   A vibrant online community for sharing recipes, tips, and personal stories.

3. **The r/carnivore Reddit Community**

   A supportive and informative forum for anyone curious about or practicing the carnivore diet.

4. **MeatRx Weekly Meetings**

   Hosted by MeatRx, these virtual meetups offer live support and advice from carnivore coaches.

Scientific References and Studies

Here are key studies and research papers that support the principles of the carnivore diet:

1. **Fatty Acid Metabolism and Cardiovascular Risk**
   - *Volek JS, Phinney SD.*
     A study exploring how low-carb, high-fat diets impact cholesterol and heart health.

2. **Nutrient Density of Animal-Based Foods**

- *Cordain L, et al.*

  This paper highlights the bioavailability of nutrients in animal products compared to plant-based foods.

3. **Effects of Red Meat Consumption on Inflammation**

   - *Turner ND, Lloyd SK.*

     Research showing how unprocessed red meat may reduce markers of inflammation when consumed in a low-carb context.

4. **Ketosis and Cognitive Function**

   - *Cunnane SC, et al.*

     A study demonstrating how ketones, derived from fat metabolism, enhance brain function and clarity.

5. **Gut Microbiome Adaptation to High-Protein Diets**
   - *Zhang C, et al.*

     Research on how the gut microbiome adapts to a high-protein, low-fiber diet, often improving digestive health.

6. **Sustainability and Environmental Impact of Livestock Farming**
   - *White RR, Hall MB.*

     A detailed analysis of the environmental benefits of regenerative farming and grass-fed livestock.